THE BATTLE FOR NORMALITY

Gerard J. M. van den Aardweg, Ph.D.

THE BATTLE FOR NORMALITY

A Guide for (Self-)Therapy for Homosexuality

IGNATIUS PRESS   SAN FRANCISCO

Cover design by Roxanne Mei Lum

© 1997 Ignatius Press, San Francisco
All rights reserved
ISBN 978-0-89870-614-7
Library of Congress catalogue number 96-76830
Printed in the United States of America ∞

To men and women tormented by homosexual emotions who do not want to live as homosexuals, who want constructive help and support, and who are forgotten, have no voice, and get no answers in our society, which recognizes only the emancipatory homosexual who wants to impose his ideology of "normality" and "unchangeability" and thus discriminates against those who know or feel that that is a sad lie.

CONTENTS

INTRODUCTION

This book gives guidelines for the therapy of homosexuality, which is essentially self-therapy. It is intended for homosexually inclined persons who want to do something about their "condition" themselves but do not have the opportunity to visit a therapist with healthy ideas on the matter. For, indeed, there are few of them. The chief reason for this is that the topic of homosexuality had been neglected or ignored at universities, and if mentioned at all, emphasis is placed on the "normality" ideology: homosexuality is just a natural sexual alternative. So there are far too few medical people, behavioral scientists, and psychotherapists who have even a rudimentary knowledge of this subject.

That the element of self-treatment predominates in any treatment of homosexuality does not as a rule mean that one can "go it alone". He who wants to overcome emotional problems needs a realistically understanding and encouraging *guide* to whom he can speak his mind, to help him discover important aspects of his emotional life and of his motivations, and to coach him in his struggle with himself. That guide need not necessarily be a professional therapist. Preferredly, he should be, but on the condition that he has healthy ideas about sexuality and morality; if not, he may do more harm than good. Occasionally, a physician or pastor with a balanced and normal personality and a capacity for realistic human insights can fill this role. If there is no one better qualified available, it may even be advisable to ask a sensible and psychologically healthy friend or relative to function as guide, as far as possible. For therapists and others

9

who may be in the position of having to support a homosexual who wants to change, this book therefore is secondarily aimed. They too cannot dispense with basic knowledge
of the homosexual condition.

I present here what I think are the essentials with regard to
insight and (self-)treatment of homosexuality, based on more
than thirty years of study and therapeutic experience with
more than three hundred clients whom I have come to know
well for several years at least and with many other ("clinical"
as well as "nonclinical", that is, socially adapted) persons with
this orientation. For research evidence relating to such factors as psychological testing and homosexuality, parental and
other intrafamily relationships, and social adaptation in childhood, I refer to my two previous books in English, especially
On the Origins and Treatment of Homosexuality (1986; see also
Homosexuality and Hope, 1985).

A Good Will

Without a strong determination, a "good will", no change is
possible. With it, improvement is certain in the majority of
cases, and in a minority, even a cure—a deep inner change in
overall neurotic emotionality and a beneficial reversal of
sexual interests—is achievable.

But who possesses that "good will"? Most afflicted persons,
including those who militantly profess their gayness, some-
how still have the desire to be normal, repressed as it may be.
Only a minority, however, really wants to change—and wants
it with some constancy, rather than as a mere impulse that is
perhaps recurring, but quickly fades away. Even among those
with the best resolution to fight their homosexuality, there is
a good deal of second thought, a hidden cherishing of the
alluring homosexual desires. So a good will is for the most

part still a weak will; and, of course, the will's weakness is easily reinforced by all the social pressures to "accept one's homosexuality". To persist in the resolution to change one must cultivate in oneself such motivators as a clear view of homosexuality as something unnatural; a sound moral and/or religious conviction; and, where applicable, the will to make the best of an existing marriage relationship that is reasonable, apart from the sexual aspect. Being well-motivated is not the same as practicing rigid self-bashing, self-hatred, or a fearful compliance with moral prescriptions simply because they are imposed by society or religion; rather, it is to have a quiet and strong feeling that homosexuality is incompatible with psychological maturity and/or moral purity, with the deepest stirrings of one's conscience, and with one's responsibility before God. To strengthen regularly one's moral resolution to fight the homosexual side of the personality is therefore crucial for a good outcome.

Results

Understandably, most of those considering treatment for their homosexuality, and other interested persons as well, are eager to know "the percentage of cures". Simple statistics, however, do not convey all the information necessary for a balanced judgment. With regard to cures, according to my experience, about 10 to 15 percent of all who entered treatment (30 percent discontinued after some months) recovered "radically". That is, after years of treatment they no longer have homosexual feelings and are normal in their heterosexuality; and their change only deepens in the course of the years. And—the third and obligatory criterion for a "radical" change—they improve greatly in terms of overall emotionality and maturity. This last aspect is essential because homosexuality is not an isolated "preference", but an expression of a specific neurotic personality. For instance, I have seen a few cases of amazingly rapid and complete change from homosexual to heterosexual interests in persons in whom an until-then dormant paranoia had got the upper hand. These are cases of real "symptom substitution", which make us aware of the clinical fact that homosexuality is much more than a functional disturbance in the sexual realm.

The majority of those who try to practice regularly the methods to be discussed here do improve, as measured after several (three to five on average) years of treatment. Their homosexual desires and fantasies become weak to nonexistent; heterosexuality comes into existence or is considerably strengthened; and their personalities become less neurotic. Some, not all, however, suffer occasional relapses (under stress, for example) of their old homosexual imagery; but if they return to the struggle the relapse usually does not last for long.

This picture is much more optimistic than emancipatory homosexuals—who have a vested interest in the dogma of the irreversibility of homosexuality—would make us believe. On the other hand, success is not so simple as some enthusiastic people from the ex-gay movement have sometimes contended. In the first place, the change process usually takes at least three to five years, in spite of all the progress that can be made within a much shorter period of time. Moreover, such change requires a persistent will, one prepared to be satisfied with small steps, small victories in everyday life, rather than expecting sudden dramatic cures. The realities of the process of change are not disappointing if we realize that the person in (self-)therapy is actually restructuring or *re-educating* a misformed and immature personality. Neither should one take the view that, when the outcome is not the complete disappearance of all homosexual inclinations, therapeutic attempts are not worth the trouble. Quite the contrary. The homosexual can only gain by the process: his sexual obsessions almost always fade away, and he becomes more happy and healthy in his outlook and, certainly, in his ways of life. Between complete cure and little or only temporary progress (which is the estimated outcome in about 20 percent of those who remain in treatment), there are many shades and grades of satisfactory improvement. But even most of those who least improve in their feelings in any case considerably restrict their homosexual contacts, and that can only be regarded as gain, in terms of both moral and physical health, as has become clear since the AIDS epidemic. (The data regarding sexually transmitted diseases and life expectancy of committed homosexuals are nothing but alarming, even if corrected for AIDS; Cameron 1992).

The case with homosexuality is, in short, as with other neuroses: phobias, obsessions, depressions, or other sexual anomalies. The most sensible thing is to try to do something about it, even if it costs energy and means giving up immediate pleasures and illusions. Most homosexuals surmise this, in fact, but because they do not want to see what is evident, some try to convince themselves that their orientation is normal and become furious if their dream, or escape from reality, is threatened. They like to exaggerate the difficulty of therapy and are certainly blind to the advantages of even slight changes for the better. But who would argue against therapies of rheumatoid diseases or cancer, even if these therapies still cannot definitively cure all categories of patients?

Successes of the Ex-Gay Movement and Other Therapies

The growing "ex-gay" movement, consisting of many loosely organized groups and organizations of those with a homosexual inclination who want to change, can point to an increasing number of profoundly improved or even cured persons. They use a mixture of psychological and Christian ideas and "methods", and in practice emphasize the element of interior struggle. The Christian believer may have an advantage in the therapy of homosexuality because his belief in the (undistorted) word of God gives him a firm orientation in life and strengthens his will to dispose of what he feels is his darker side and to long for moral purity. Despite some imbalances, such as an occasional overenthusiastic and somewhat premature tendency to "witness" and to expect "miracles" too easily, there is something we must learn from this Christian movement, a lesson that is learned in private practice, too: *the therapy of homosexuality is a psychological, spiritual, and moral affair*, even more so than the therapies of a number of other neuroses. Conscience is involved, as are man's spiritual efforts, which teach him that giving in to homosexuality and to the homosexual lifestyle is irreconcilable with real peace of mind and being authentically religious. So many homosexuals try obsessively to reconcile the irreconcilable and imagine that they can be devout as well as homosexually active. The artificiality and self-deception of such attempts are apparent, however; they end up living as homosexuals and forgetting about Christianity or creating their own homosexuality-compatible version of Christianity to cover up their conscience. As for the therapy of homosexuality, the combination of spiritual-moral elements and psychological insights in all probability offers the most fruitful perspectives.

I do not wish to give the impression that in presenting the basic insights into homosexuality and its therapy, I am thereby invalidating other insights and methods. To my mind, the similarities in modern psychological theories and therapies are much greater than their differences. Notably, the basic insight that homosexuality is a problem of gender identification is shared by almost all of them. Moreover, therapeutic methods may differ in practice less than it might seem if one merely looks at the textbooks. There certainly is a good deal of overlap in methods. This said, and with great respect for all my colleagues who work in this field who try to see through the riddles of homosexuality and to help the troubled find their true identity, I offer what I think is the best theoretical combination of the various theories and insights, leading to the most effective methods of (self-)treatment. The more accurate our observations and conclusions are, the better the self-insight of the concerned homosexual person, and how far he can recover ultimately depends on *his* self-insight.

PART ONE

INSIGHTS

HOMOSEXUALITY: AN OVERVIEW

Insights in Brief

In order to sharpen the reader's understanding of the view expounded here, let us first highlight its distinguishing points. What is central here is the notion of the homosexual's unconscious self-pity. This strong habit is not willful, but autonomous. It propels "masochistic" behavior. The homosexual wish itself is embedded in this unconscious self-pity, as are his *feelings of gender inferiority*. This view harmonizes the notions and behavioral observations of Alfred Adler (1930; that inferiority complex and compensation wishes aim at "reparation" of inferiority), Austrian-American psychoanalyst Edmund Bergler (1957; homosexuality as "psychic masochism"), and Dutch psychiatrist Johan Arndt (1961; concept of compulsive self-pity).

Secondly, by his *masculinity/feminity inferiority complex* or *gender inferiority complex*, the homosexual partly remains "a child", "a teenager"; this observation is known as *psychic infantilism*. This Freudian notion has been emphasized for homosexuality by Wilhelm Stekel (1922) and is in line with more modern notions about "the inner child of the past" (American child psychiatrist Missildine 1963; Harris 1973; and others).

Thirdly, more or less specific parental attitudes and parent–

child relationships may predispose one to the development of a homosexual gender inferiority complex. Yet the lack of same-sex group adaptation weighs even more heavily as a predisposing factor. Traditional psychoanalysis reduced all emotional malformation and neurosis to disturbed parent–child relationships; without denying the great importance of child–parent interactions, the final determining factor generally lies more, however, in the adolescent's self-image in terms of gender, *as compared with same-sex peers*. Herein, our view synchronizes with such neo-psychoanalysts as Karen Horney (1950) and Johan Arndt (1961) and self-image theorists as Carl Rogers (1951) and others.

Fourthly, fear of the opposite sex is frequent (psychoanalysts such as Ferenczi [1914, 1950]; Fenichel [1945]) but is not a primary cause of homosexual inclinations. Rather, this fear is a symptom of gender inferiority feelings; these indeed can be activated by members of the opposite sex, who are perceived as expecting sex roles the homosexual feels unable to perform.

Fifthly, giving in to homosexual wishes creates a *sexual addiction*. Persons who have reached this stage have essentially two problems: their gender inferiority complex and a relatively autonomous sexual addiction (a situation comparable to that of a neurotic with a drinking problem). American psychiatrist Lawrence J. Hatterer (1980) has written on this double syndrome of "pleasure addiction".

Sixthly, in (self-)therapy, a special role is given to self-humor. Here we have the notions of self-irony of Adler, of "hyperdramatization" of Arndt, and more or less those of behavior therapist Stampfl's (1967) "implosion", and Austrian psychiatrist Viktor Frankl's (1975) "paradoxical intention".

Lastly, inasmuch as homosexual desires are rooted in self-centeredness or immature "egophilia"—the term comes from Murray (1953)—(self-)therapy emphasizes the acquisition of those human and moral virtues that have a "de-egocentrizing" effect and enhance the capacity to love.

Not Normal

It is obvious that the vast majority of people still think ho-mosexuality—being sexually attracted to members of one's own sex, along with an at least substantial reduction of het-erosexual interests—is abnormal. I use the word "still", for this is a fact in spite of a prolonged bombardment of normal-ity propaganda by the ignorant and slavishly trendy social and political ideologists who rule the media, politics, and a great part of the academic world. If the social elite of this time have lost their common sense, not so the great mass of people, who perhaps can be forced to accept social measures coming from the "equal rights" ideology of homosexuality emancipators, but not to change the simple observation that something must be wrong with people who, although physi-ologically men and women, do not feel attracted to the obvi-ously natural objects of the propagation-directed sex instinct. To the bewildered question of many on why it is possible that "educated people" could believe that homosexuality is normal, perhaps the best answer is George Orwell's saying that there are things "so foolish that only intellectuals could believe them". The phenomenon is not new: many a noted scientist began "believing" the "correct" racist ideology in the Germany of the thirties. For many the herd-instinct, a weakness of character, and an anxiety "to belong" make them sacrifice their independent judgment.

If someone is starving while his feelings fearfully reject the object of the hunger drive, food, we know the person suffers from a disturbance (anorexia nervosa). If someone cannot feel compassion at the sight of those suffering, or worse, even enjoys their suffering, yet becomes sentimental at the sight of an abandoned kitten, we recognize an emotional disturbance (psychopathy). And so on. However, if an adult lacks the capacity for erotic arousal by the opposite sex, while he obsessively chases same-sex partners, this failure of the sexual instinct is considered "healthy". Would then pedophilia likewise be normal (as pedophilia advocates already say)? Exhibitionism? Gerontophilia (being attracted to elderly people in the absence of normal heterosexuality)? Fetishism (a woman's shoe causes sexual excitement, the body of the woman indifference)? Voyeurism? I will skip over other, more bizarre and, fortunately, more rare deviations.

Militant homosexuals try to force on the public the idea that they are normal by playing the role of victim of discrimination, thus appealing to the sentiments of compassion and justice and to the instinct of protection of the weak, instead of convincing by way of argument and rational proof. This in itself shows that they are aware of the logical weakness of their position. Their vehement emotionality is an attempt to overcompensate for their want of rational grounds. With people of this mind-set, matter-of-fact discussion is nearly impossible, for they refuse to consider any view that does not fully endorse their normality dogma. But do they, deep down, really believe it themselves?

Such militants may succeed well in transferring their view of themselves as martyrs to others—their mothers, for instance. In a German town I met a group of parents of avowed homosexuals, who had united to fight for their sons' "rights". They were not less indignant and overemotional in their irrational argumentation than their sons themselves. Some mothers behaved as if their favorite baby's life was endangered if one merely contended that homosexuality is a neurotic condition.

The Role of Self-Labeling

This brings us to the psychologically dangerous *decision* to identify oneself as a different species of man: "I *am* a homosexual." As if the essence of that existence were different from that of heterosexuals. It may give a sense of relief after a period of struggle and worry, but at the same time it is defeatist. The self-identified homosexual takes on the role of the definitive outsider. It is, in fact, a *tragic* role. Quite different from a sober and realistic self-appraisal: I have these fantasies and feelings, still I resist taking on the role and identity of "homosexual".

That role brings certain rewards, to be sure. It makes one feel at home among fellow homosexuals. It temporarily takes away the tension of having to fight homosexual impulses, and yields the emotional gratifications of feeling unique and tragic—however unconscious that may be—and, of course, of having sexual adventures. Recalling her discovery of the lesbian subculture, an ex-lesbian writes about the "sense of belonging" it gave her: "As though I had come home. I had found my true peer group [recall the homosexual's childhood drama of feeling the outsider]. Looking back now, I see how needy we all were—a group of misfits who had finally found a niche in life" (Howard 1991, 117). The coin has another side, however. Real happiness, let alone inner peace, is never found that way. Restlessness will increase, as will the feeling of an inner void. Conscience will send out its disquieting and persistent signals. For it is a false "self" the unhappy person has identified with. The door to the homosexual "way of life" has opened. Initially, it is a seducing dream; in time it turns out to be a terrible illusion. "Being a homosexual" means leading an unreal life, ever farther away from one's real person.

"Self-labeling" is greatly stimulated by the propaganda that repeats that many people simply "are" homosexual. But homosexual interests are often, perhaps usually, not constant. There are highs and lows; periods when the person has more or less heterosexual feelings may alternate with fits of homosexuality. Certainly, many youngsters and young adults who did not cultivate the self-image of "being homosexual" have thereby prevented themselves from developing a full-fledged homosexual orientation. Self-labeling, on the other hand, reinforces the homosexual side, especially when it is only in its beginnings, and starves the heterosexual component. It is important to recognize that about half of homosexual men can be regarded as bisexuals and the proportion among women is even larger.

2

DEVELOPMENT OF HOMOSEXUALITY

Homosexuality in the Genes? In the Brain?

"In the hormones?" is not added to this heading because, except for an occasional reference (e.g., the rat studies by the East German Dörner—which are irrelevant for humans, besides being quantitatively incorrect), the trend to look for hormonal evidence as proof of a specific homosexual "nature" has subsided. There appears to be no ground for a hormonal theory. We must notice, however, that those who would normalize homosexuality have for decades propagandistically exploited every shred of hormonal evidence, however vague it was. They tried to give the impression that "science" had thus proved the normalcy of homosexuality and that those who disagreed were following obsolete theories. In that respect, nothing much has changed, only that by now some highly ambiguous findings in the brain of deceased homosexuals, or suggestions of peculiarities in the sex-linked chromosomes of a specific group of them must serve as "scientific proof".

If some biological factor were found to be narrowly correlated with homosexuality, that would, nevertheless, be no argument at all for its normality. Neither would it of necessity be a direct cause; it might as easily be a consequence of this orientation. It is, however, still a big "if". The overall evidence in the biological field points to nonphysiological, nonbiological causation.

Recently, two studies were widely published with the suggestion that "there probably is a biologic-hereditary cause." Hamer et al. (1993) found indications of a similarity in a small part of the X chromosome (inheritable from the mother) in two-thirds of a group of homosexual men when compared with their homosexual brothers. Does that mean that they found a gene that causes homosexuality? Not by a long shot. As most geneticists agree, such results must be found again and again before a genetic correlation can be established. Similar "discoveries" of a gene for schizophrenia, manic-depressive psychosis, and alcoholism (even delinquency!) have silently died away from want of subsequent confirmation. Besides, this study is only about some genetic factor in the small segment of the population of male homosexuals who happen to have homosexual brothers (assuming that the criteria for being "homosexual" used are acceptable, which is often a point of debate in this type of study), i.e., in at most 6 percent (two-thirds of at most 10 percent) of homosexual males. I say "at most" because the group under study might be representative only for committed homosexuals with similarly feeling brothers, since it had been collected by means of advertising in homosexual publications. If confirmed, this study would not in itself prove a genetic cause, as closer inspection of the gene might reveal it to be anything: a trait of physical similarity to the mother, a temperamental trait, such as a proneness to anxiety, and so on. One could then suppose that certain mothers or fathers would raise a son with such a characteristic in a less masculine mode. Or that boys with the gene would be predisposed to maladjustment to their same-sex peer group (if the gene were linked to fearfulness, for example). The gene would determine nothing by itself. That it is associated with sexuality as such is already unlikely because homosexuals—or the small proportion with this gene—would then possess particular hormonal and/or brain factors, and this has never been demonstrated.

William Byne (1994) raises an interesting additional question. Similarity between homosexual sons and their mothers in the molecular sequence in the X-chromosome area under study, he observes, does not point to one identical gene for all these men, for it is not shown that they share one and the same molecular sequence. (One pair of brothers could resemble their mother in eye color, another pair, the shape of the nose, and so on).

The improbability of a causative or predisposing *sexual* gene arises from two facts: (1) there is no pattern of Mendelian inheritance in families of homosexuals, and (2) results of studies with twins are more in line with "environmental" than genetic explanations. Here too, curious things have occurred. Kallmann reported in 1952 that in 100 percent of identical twins of whom one was a homosexual, the twin brother was homosexual too, compared with only 11 percent for nonidentical twins of whom one was a homosexual. Didn't that suggest heredity? No, for Kallmann's sample afterward turned out to have been highly biased and unrepresentative, and it soon became clear that there were many nonhomosexuals among otherwise selected identical twins. Recently, Bailey and Pillard (1991) found a homosexuality concordance of 52 percent for identical male twins and 22 percent for nonidentical, *but* 9 percent of (other) homosexuals had a homosexual brother and even 11 percent had an *adopted* brother who was homosexual. First then, in only half of the cases could a homosexuality-related genetic factor have been decisive, indicating that it could hardly be a determining cause. Second, the differences between the nonidentical twin pairs on the one hand, and homosexuals and other brothers (including adoptive brothers) on the other (22 percent, 9 percent, and 11 percent, respectively), point to nongenetic causes, as nonidentical twins differ genetically as much as any siblings. The psychology of twins gives the better explanation for the observed relationships. There are other reservations as well; for instance, other studies report lower identical-twin concordance for homosexuality, and the samples of most studies are not representative for the overall homosexual population.

Back to the Hamer study: it is much too early, in fact, for genetic speculations because, among other reasons, we do not know if the speculative "gene" would not also be present in heterosexual brothers of homosexuals and in the heterosexual population. Perhaps the most lethal criticism against the study has been raised by Risch, who devised the statistical test that provided Hamer with his results. According to Risch, the statistical requirements for the test were not met in this particular group (Risch et al. 1993). Hamer, despite fueling the notion that his findings "suggest" a genetic influence, nevertheless himself states that it would be "likely" that homosexuality could also arise from "environmental causes" (Hamer et al. 1993). The problem is, however, that such "suggestions" are publicized as near-proof.

In *Science* magazine, LeVay had reported two years before (1991) that a group of homosexual men who had died of AIDS had smaller nuclei in a certain region of the brain (the anterior hypothalamus) compared to nonhomosexual men who had died of the same disease. Around the globe the question was raised: "A neurological basis for homosexuality?" Not exactly. The overlap between the homosexuals and the controls in nucleus size was considerable, so that this factor could not account for a minority of the homosexuals. Further, the assumption of LeVay that this brain region was a sexual center has been disproved; and criticisms have been made of his method of tissue preparation (Byne and Parsons 1993). There is more. He left out a group of homosexual patients because they had too much brain pathology. Indeed, AIDS is known to change brain anatomy, as it also causes alterations in the DNA. (Another possible explanation of the genetic findings of Hamer et al.: Did they, by recruiting their subjects among active homosexuals, leave out those infected by HIV or other sexually transmitted viruses?) In their thorough review of homosexuality and "biological" factors, Byne and Parsons notice that the AIDS history of homosexuals differs from that of heterosexual intravenous drug addicts, who on the average die sooner than contaminated homosexuals and are likely to have had other medical treatments.

Suppose homosexuals did show similarities in specific brain regions. Would homosexual pedophiliacs then have their own specific brain site? And heterosexual pedophiliacs? Homosexual and heterosexual masochists, and sadists, each their own? Exhibitionists? Voyeurists? Homosexual and heterosexual fetishists? Homosexual and heterosexual transvestites? Transsexuals? Persons sexually aroused by animals, or with even more aberrant preferences?

The improbability of sexual orientation having a genetic origin is manifested, moreover, by behavioral patterns. It is known, for example, that even in persons with deviant chromosomes, sexual orientation depends primarily on the sex role in which the child has been reared. And would successful psychotherapy, resulting in the radical reorientation of homosexuals, which indubitably does occur, then cause changes in the genes? Unlikely.

As to possible differences in brain anatomy between homosexuals and heterosexuals, we cannot rule out that certain brain structures could change *as a consequence* of behavior habits. Why then did LeVay, who aptly wrote that his results "did not allow one to draw conclusions" in another place in his article still say that they "suggested" a biological substrate for homosexuality (and naturally this "suggestion" in thin air was quickly picked up by the homosexuality-normalizing media)? It is not being too suspicious to conjecture that emancipatory homosexual politics have to do with that. LeVay is a professed homosexual. The strategy of the emancipators is to create the impression that probably there are biological causes; we do not exactly know them as yet, but there are interesting/promising indications. This strategy supports the "you are born that way" ideology. It is helpful for the normalization cause, because if politicians and lawmakers are brought to believe that science is on its way to proving that homosexuality is just a natural variant, that will easily translate into new homosexual rights legislation. *Science*, like other homosexuality-friendly periodicals, is inclined to support the normalization ideology. One can sense it by the way the editor describes the report by Hamer et al.: "seemingly objective". "It is indeed still a long way to a definitive proof, yet . . .", in short, suggestive emancipatory rhetoric. Commenting on Hamer's article in a letter, the famous French geneticist Prof. Lejeune (1993) even stated bluntly that "were it not for the fact that this study was about homosexuality, it would not have been accepted for publication because of its very disputable methodology and statistical insufficiency."[1]

It is a pity that few investigators who report this kind of data seem to know the *history* of the various biological "discoveries" concerning homosexuals. We recall the fate of the "finding" of Steinach, who, long before World War II, thought he had demonstrated specific changes in the testicles of male homosexuals. Many in those times had based their ideas on a biological cause on his publications. Only after many years did it become apparent that his results had not been valid.

[1] Further, concerning Hamer's data, *Scientific American* (Nov. 1995), p. 26, reports on a comprehensive study by G. Ebers, who could not find a linkage between homosexuality and markers on either the X or other chromosomes.

Not only is public opinion manipulated by such premature, suggestive publishing, it is equally deplorable that well-intentioned homosexuals who seek the truth, and those who want to fight their penchant, are also easily discouraged by it. Therefore, let us not be deceived.

Irreversibly Programmed in the First Years of Life?

The infantilism of the homosexual complex generally stems from adolescence, to a lesser degree from earlier childhood. These are the periods to which the homosexual person is fixated. It is not during early childhood, however, that the homosexual's fate is sealed, as is often contended by, among others, emancipatory homosexuals. This theory helps to justify such indoctrination of children in sex education as: "A number of you are this way and must live according to your nature." Early fixation of sexual orientation is also a favorite concept in older psychoanalytic theories. These contend that, by the age of three or four, one's basic personality is firmly formed, once and for all.

A homosexual man imagined, after hearing such a theory, that his inclinations had already been imprinted in the embryonic stage, because his mother was wishing for a girl and therefore at that tender stage would have rejected him, a boy. Irrespective of the fact that an embryo's perception is still restricted to sensations more primitive than the awareness of not being wanted, such a theory has a fatalistic flaw and reinforces the person's self-dramatization. Besides, if one relied on the memories of his youth, the period of neurotization of this man had rather clearly been adolescence. There is an element of truth in early-childhood theories, though. It is likely, for instance, that this man's mother had seen him, from his first years onward, more as a girl than a boy and that she unconsciously was influenced by that wish in how she treated him. While character traits and attitudes may indeed take shape even in the first years of life, this is not so for the homosexual inclination itself, nor the specific gender inferiority complex from which it springs.

That sexual interests are not unshakably anchored in early childhood may be illustrated by the findings of Gundlach and Riess (1967): in a large group of lesbians, these women were found to be significantly less often the eldest from families with five or more children, as compared to heterosexual women. This suggests that the decisive turn in the lesbian development does not take place before, say, six or seven years of age at its earliest, and probably later, because it is only then that a firstborn girl finds herself in the position that her chance of becoming a lesbian is enhanced (in case she has fewer than five siblings) or lowered (if five or more younger brothers and sisters are born). Similarly, a study on homosexual men from families with more than four children reported that they ranked more often than to be expected among the younger half of the children (Van Lennep et al. 1954).

Moreover, even of extraordinarily feminine boys—perhaps the group with the highest risk of becoming homosexual because of their liability to contract a masculinity inferiority complex—more than 30 percent did not develop homosexual fantasies in adolescence (Green 1985), while 20 percent moved back and forth on the sexual-interest continuum during that phase of development (Green 1987). Looking back on their early childhood, some homosexuals—not all, to be sure—can see the signs (cross-gender dressing, cross-gender games or preferences) that indicated their later orientation, but that does not imply that from these signs one can predict homosexuality in an individual child. They indicate a higher than normal chance, but not irreversible fate.

Psychological Childhood Factors

If an unprejudiced person with absolutely no idea of the origins of homosexuality would have to decide, on the basis of the best-established available facts, where to look for the solution of the question of cause(s), he would end up relying on psychological childhood factors. Yet the prevalent idea that one is born a homosexual makes it hard to believe that "psychology" and "childhood" would provide the keys to understanding. For instance, how could a man whose whole demeanor is thoroughly effeminate, to the smallest details of his gestures, his voice, have been born normal? And as for homosexuals themselves, don't they experience their desires as the urging of some instinct, as the expression of their "true selves"? Does not the very idea that they could feel like heterosexuals strike them as unnatural?

Yet appearances can be deceiving. Effeminate men need not be homosexuals, in the first place. Moreover, effeminacy is best understood as "learned" behavior. We usually do not realize to what extent habits of behaving, interests, and attitudes may be learned, most of the time through *imitation*. We can recognize the region of the country a person comes from by the melody of his speech, his pronunciation, often too by his gestures and ways. It is also quite possible to recognize members of the same family by their shared characteristics, manners, specific humor, by many behavioral aspects that are clearly not inherited. Returning to effeminacy, we note that, in general, boys in the Latin part of Europe are reared to be somewhat "softer", more "feminine" one might say, than in the northwestern part. Boys from northern countries may be irritated when they see Spanish or Italian boys combing their hair elaborately at the edge of a swimming pool, looking a long time in the mirror, wearing necklaces, etc. Likewise, sons of laborers are generally more rough and tough, more "masculine" than sons of intellectuals, musicians, and, in former days, aristocrats. The latter teach and show by their example more "refined"—read "feminine"—ways. Let us pursue this line of thinking: Who would believe a boy raised by his mother and an aunt, with no father around, and who, in addition, is treated by his lonely mother as her "girl-friend", would become a firm, masculine type? Upon analysis of childhood relationships, it becomes clear that many effeminate homosexuals lived with too great a dependency on their mother *in the absence of a father*, physically or *psychologically* (e.g., a weak man dominated by his wife or one who did not play much of the father role toward the boy).

The portrait of the demasculinizing mother has a lot of variants: the overcaring or overprotective mother who worried too much about the boy's health; the domineering mother who subjugated the boy into the role of servant or favorite friend; the sentimental or self-dramatizing mother who unconsciously saw the boy as the girl she would have liked to have had (e.g., after the death of a baby girl before the boy's birth); the older mother who could not have children when she was young; the grandmother who educated the boy she saw as needing protection after his own mother left him, or died; the child-mother who saw in her male baby more of a doll than a boy; the foster mother who treated the boy too much as a helpless and love-deprived child; and so on. Usually, background factors like these can be found in the childhood of effeminate—and other—male homosexuals, and there is no need to resort to heredity to explain the son's feminine attitudes and behaviors.

A conspicuously effeminate homosexual who had been mother's favorite, while his only brother had been a "father's boy", told me that he had always been kept in the role of his mother's "maidservant", her "page boy". He combed her hair, accompanied her when she bought a dress, and so on. Since the men's world was more or less closed to him due to his father's rather uninterested manner toward him, his world was that of his mother and his aunts. This is the reason why his imitation instinct remained directed to older females; for instance, he discovered that he could emulate them in embroidery and that he received their admiration for that. Normally, a boy's imitation instinct, after about three years, spontaneously directs itself to male models: father, brothers, uncles, teachers, and, in puberty, to other male heroes. The imitation need of girls directs itself to female models. This is best seen as an *inborn* sex-linked trait. Why some boys will imitate members of the opposite sex more than those of the same sex is due to two factors: they are pressured into the opposite-sex role, and they are discouraged from imitating their father, brothers, or other males. *The natural course of the instinct to imitate same-sex behavior is thwarted if there is a lack of encouragement in combination with too much reward for imitating behavior of the opposite sex.* In the case just mentioned, the boy felt happy and secure with the attention and admiration of his mother and aunts, while he felt he didn't have a chance in the world of his brother and his father. He developed the *personality traits* and attitudes of a "mama's boy"; he was obsequious, tried to please everyone, especially older women; like his mother, he was quickly moved to tears and sentimental, talkative in the manner of an old woman, and easily hurt and insulted. It is of importance to notice that the femininity of such men has an "old-womanish" quality; although it is deeply ingrained role-playing, it is merely a pseudo-femininity. It is not only a flight from male behavior out of fear of failure, but also a form of infantile attention-seeking, an enjoyment in the admiration this posing as the "woman" may bring from the significant women in their environment. This is most visible in trans-sexual types and woman impersonators.

Traumatization and habits of behavior

No doubt, the element of *traumatization* plays a substantial role in the psychological malformation underlying homo-sexuality (particularly with regard to same-sex adaptation, see below). The "maidservant" man I just discussed of course re-membered having longed for the same attention from his fa-ther that his brother, in his view, did receive. But his habits and interests could not be explained as being merely a flight from the men's world. There is often an interplay between two factors: habit formation—in fact, malformation—and traumatization, feeling unable to cope with the same-sex world. It is necessary to stress this habit factor, apart from the frustration factor, for an effective therapy must not try only to overcome the neurotic consequences of traumatization, but also to re-form learned cross-gender habits. In addition, exclusive attention to the traumatization element, however powerful that may have been, may reinforce the self-victim-izing tendency of homosexually inclined persons and give rise to "blaming" (insofar as this term might be used here at all) the same-sex parent alone. For instance, it is not always a father's "fault" that he did not pay sufficient attention to the boy. Sometimes a homosexual's father will complain that his wife was so possessive of their son that he felt he could not interfere. Indeed, many parents of homosexuals had serious marriage problems.

As for the feminine behavior of male homosexuals and the masculine of lesbians, the clinical fact is that many of them have positively been reared in a role that was to a de-gree different from the role of other children of their sex. That they later adhered to that role is often indeed the di-rect result of a lack of positive encouragement on the part of the same-sex parent. The common denominator, how-ever, of the inner attitude of many (but not all!) mothers of homosexual men is that they *did not view and/or treat this son as a "real man"*. And, although apparently to a lesser degree, some fathers of lesbians did not see or treat their daughter sufficiently as a "real girl", but sometimes more as their favorite comrade, or as a son.

It should be noted that the role of the parent of the opposite sex is just as important as that of the same-sex parent. Many male homosexuals, for instance, had an overprotecting, anxious, worrying, or dominant mother, or one who overly admired and pampered them. Her son was "the nice boy", "the obedient boy", "the well-behaved boy", and very often, a boy who was retarded in psychological development, who had been kept "a baby" for too long. And the later homosexual man has partly remained that particular mother's boy. But a dominant mother, if she sees her boy as a "real man" and wants to make a man of him, will not produce a "sissy" boy. The same applies to father–daughter relationships. It is the dominant (overprotective, overanxious, and so on) mother who did not know how to make a man of her boy, who unwittingly contributed to his psychological malformation. Often, she did not have a good idea of what it means to make a man out of a boy, perhaps lacking good examples in her own family. She was anxious to make a well-behaved model boy out of him or to attach him to herself when she was lonely and very insecure (like the mother who took her son with her in bed until his twelfth year).

In short, the study of homosexuality shows the importance of parents' having healthy notions and habits with regard to masculinity and femininity. In the majority of cases, however, it is the *combination* of the attitudes of both parents that prepares the ground for a homosexual development (van den Aardweg 1984).

One may ask if feminine traits in homosexual men and masculine in lesbians would then be a prerequisite for homosexuality. The majority of prehomosexual boys are indeed more or less effeminate, as most—not all—prehomosexual girls have slight or more marked masculine traits. However, neither this "femininity" nor "masculinity" is crucial. It is, as we shall see, the child's *self-perception as masculine or feminine* that makes all the difference. Even in cases of strong effeminate behavior in preadolescent boys, called the "sissy syndrome", no more than two-thirds developed homosexual fantasies in adolescence and some lost their conspicuous effeminacy after becoming adults (Green 1985, 1987). This result, by the way, synchronizes with the notion that in most cases it is during the periods of preadolescence and adolescence that a homosexual fixation takes place, not early childhood.

Atypical cases

While poor relationships with parents of the same sex, often accompanied by unhealthy attachment bonds with parents of the opposite sex (especially for male homosexuals), are a common childhood experience for homosexual persons, they are by no means a universal phenomenon. Some male homosexuals had good relationships with their fathers, felt loved and esteemed by them; and some lesbians had good mother relationships (Howard 1991, 83). But even such largely positive relationships can play a role in the development of homosexuality.

For example, a young homosexual, slightly feminine in behavior, had been chiefly reared by his affectionate and appreciating father. He remembered that as a child he wanted to go home as soon as possible after school, where he felt uneasy and could not cope with his peers (the decisive factor!). "Home" for him did not mean, as one would expect, being with his mother, but with his father, whose favorite he was

and by whom he felt protected. Nor was his father the familiar weak type, with whom he would not have been able to
"identify"—on the contrary. It was his mother who was the
weak and timid personality and who did not play a significant
role in his childhood. His father was a manly, aggressive type
whom he admired. The important point seems to have been
that his father imposed on him the role of a girl, and of a
weakling, as if he had no strength to defend himself in this
world. His father dominated him in a friendly way, so he was
really close to him. His father's attitude created, or helped to
create, in him the view of himself as defenseless and helpless,
not manly and "strong". As an adult, this man kept clinging to
fatherly friends for support. His erotic interest, however, focused on young men, not on older, fatherly types.

Likewise, a seemingly manly homosexual man of about
forty-five could not detect the slightest problem in his childhood relationship with his father. His father had been his
friend, his coach in sports, and a good masculine model in his
work and social relationships. Why then did he not "identify"
with his father's masculinity? The problem lay with his
mother. She was proud and dissatisfied with his father's social
achievements. More intelligent and from a higher social level
than her husband, who was a working man, she often humiliated him with her sharp criticisms and contemptuous wit.
The son had always felt sorry for him. He *did* identify with his
father, but not with his manly behavior, because he had been
taught by his mother to see himself as different from his father. As his mother's favorite, he was to be the one who would
compensate her for her disappointment in her husband.
Manly qualities had never been stimulated in him; except for
the quality of achieving socially, these were regarded as inferior. He had to be sophisticated and brilliant. Despite his
healthy bond with his father, he had ever felt ashamed for his
own masculinity. I think his mother's scorn and her disrespect

for the role of the father and for his authority had primarily been responsible for the son's difficulty in feeling manly pride.

This type of motherly attitude has been seen as "castrative" to a boy's manliness, and we can agree with that, assuming it is not meant in the literal Freudian sense of a mother who wants to cut off her husband's or son's penis. Likewise, a husband who humiliates his wife in front of his children damages their respect for women in general. His daughter may refer his lack of esteem for the other sex to herself. Fathers, by a negative attitude toward the feminine sex, may therefore inspire in a daughter a negative and rejecting attitude toward her own feminity. Mothers, by a negative attitude toward the masculine role of their husband, or sometimes toward masculinity in general, may facilitate a son's negative view of his own masculinity.

There are homosexually oriented men who felt their fathers' affection, but missed their fatherly protection. One father who felt unable to cope with life leaned on his son in times of trouble, a practice the son felt as too heavy a burden, for he wanted support from a strong father himself. The roles of parent and child seem reversed in those cases, as with those women with lesbian inclinations who as girls felt they had to play the mother role with respect to their own mothers. A girl in such a relationship would then feel that she could not get her mother's necessary understanding for her own normal problems and would miss her mother's encouragement of her feminine self-confidence, which is of such importance during puberty.

Other factors: Peer relationships

The statistical evidence regarding the homosexual's childhood parental relationships is convincing. Repeatedly, it has been found (in non-Western cultures as well) that apart from frequent unhealthy mother-bonds, homosexual men had poor relationships with their fathers, and lesbians had less familiarity with their mothers compared to heterosexuals and heterosexual neurotics. Nevertheless, it must be remembered that parental and educational factors are preparatory, predisposing, but not decisive. The ultimate prime cause of homosexuality in men is not, for instance, a pathological mother attachment nor rejection by the father, no matter how often evidence of such situations is found in the analysis of the afflicted person's youth years. Lesbianism is not the direct result of a feeling of rejection by the mother, notwithstanding the frequency of this childhood factor. (We can see this easily if we think of the many heterosexual adults who in their childhood were also rejected by a same-sex parent, even abandoned. Among criminals and delinquent adolescents, many suffered from that situation, and one finds it often enough in heterosexual neurotics too.)

The strongest association, then, is not found between homosexuality and father–child and mother–child relationships, but between homosexuality and *"peer relationships"*. (For statistical tables and overviews, see van den Aardweg 1986, 78, 80; Nicolosi 1991, 63). Regrettably, the impact of traditional psychoanalytic notions, with their almost exclusive interest in parent–child interactions, is still so heavy that few theorists have taken this objective finding seriously enough. It should be made the *prime suspect* in any explanation of homosexuality for our imaginary unbiased person who is after insight into its causes.

Peer relationships, in turn, can significantly influence the factor that is of paramount importance: the teenager's *self-view as to his masculinity or her femininity*. In a girl, for example, apart from such factors as a lack of security in her relation with the mother, being the favorite of the father (or, on the contrary, being neglected by the father), quite different things can influence that self-view: teasing by peers, feelings of inferiority in relation to her siblings; physical clumsiness; "ugliness", that is, the perception of not being pretty or attractive in the eyes of boys during puberty; or having been viewed by family members as being boyish ("you are just like your uncle"). Such negative experiences can lead to the complex examined below.

The Masculinity/Femininity Inferiority Complex

"The American idea of *masculinity*: There are few things under heaven more difficult to understand or, when I was younger, more difficult to forgive." With these words, the black homosexual author James Baldwin (1985, 678) expressed his frustration over his perception of himself as a failure with respect to that trait. He scorned what he could not realize himself. He felt the *victim* of this forced-upon masculinity, an outcast; in short, inferior. His view of "American masculinity" was distorted by this frustration. Certainly, there are exaggerated forms—macho behavior or criminal "hardness"—that may be taken by the immature as being really "masculine", but there also exist a healthy masculine courage, sportsmanship, competitiveness, and persistence, which are the antipode of weakness, softness to oneself, an "old womanish" demeanor, or effeminacy. Baldwin as a youth felt he lacked that positive virtue of manliness in coping with his peers, perhaps more painfully at high school, during puberty: "I was physically a target. . . . It worked against me, y'know, to be the brightest boy in class and the smallest boy in class. And I suffered." He was teased, nicknamed "bug eyes" and "sissy", and could not defend himself. His father could not encourage him, being a weak personality; Baldwin was brought up by his mother and grandmother, a protected child in whose life the manly element was too absent. His feeling distant from the world of manhood was aggravated when he learned that his father was not his biological father. His experience could be summed up as "The other boys, who are more manly, are against me." His being called "sissy" reflects this, for the term does not mean being seen as a real girl, it means *not being a normal man, being an inferior man*. It is nearly synonymous with being a weakling, one who cries easily, as girls do, who does not fight but flees. Baldwin may have blamed "American" masculinity for his feelings, but, in fact, male homosexuals throughout the world criticize the masculinity of the culture they live in, for they invariably feel inferior in just that respect. Lesbians for the same reason may be contemptuous of what they, distortedly because of their negative experiences, see as "that prescribed femininity: dolling yourself up, having to be interested only in trivial household things, having to be the attractive, sweet girl", as one Dutch lesbian woman put it. Feeling less masculine or feminine than others is the specific inferiority complex of homosexually oriented people.

As a matter of fact, prehomosexuals not only feel "different"—which translates into "inferior"—but also often do have a less boyish (girlish), less manly (womanly) demeanor than their same-sex peers and have less gender-typical interests. They have atypical *habits*, or *personality traits*, as a result of their upbringing and parental relationships. It has been shown over and over again that a lack of masculine traits in childhood and adolescence—such as being more fearful of physical injury than other boys, being less aggressive, not participating in the favorite games of boys (soccer in Europe and Latin America, baseball in the U.S.)—is the first and foremost fact that is associated with male homosexuality. Female homosexuals generally have less "feminine" interests as compared with other girls (for statistics, van den Aardweg 1986). Hockenberry and Billingham (1987) rightly concluded that "it may be the *absence of masculine traits rather than the presence of feminine traits* that is the stronger and most influential variable for a future (male) homosexual." A boy whose father was hardly present in his life and whose mother was perhaps too much, cannot develop his masculine side. Some variant of this rule has been operative in the youth of most male homosexuals. Characteristically, as boys, homosexual men did not imagine themselves as future policemen, did not prefer boys' games, did not imagine themselves as sports figures, were considered "sissies", did not read adventure stories, and so on (Hockenberry and Billingham 1987). As a consequence, they felt inferior in their peer group. As girls, lesbians characteristically felt inferior in femininity. Feeling "ugly" often contributed to such a self-perception, and this is understandable. The preadolescent and adolescent stages together are primarily when the young person develops his self-image regarding his position among his same-sex peers: Do I belong to them? *Comparison of himself* with the others determines his self-image with regard to gender characteristics more than anything else. A young homosexually oriented man boasted that he had never felt inferior and that his outlook had always been cheerful. The only thing that worried him, he thought, was the lack of social acceptance of his orientation. After some self-searching, he confirmed that he indeed had been carefree in his childhood, feeling secure with both his parents (who overprotected him), but only until adolescence. From childhood on, he had had three friends. He had felt increasingly abandoned by them because they grew closer to each other than to him. Their interests developed in the direction of "rougher" sports, their conversations were about men's things—girls, sports—and he could not catch up with them. He tried to make himself "count" to them, playing the funny boy who made everyone laugh, in order to get attention. He had never wanted to admit it to himself, but his adolescence was marked by spells of sadness and by inner loneliness.

Here we have the crucial point: he felt terribly unmanly in their company. At home, he had been a protected child; he had been raised as a "quiet, well-behaved" boy; his mother had always been proud of his good manners. He never quarreled; "You must always keep peace" was his mother's favorite advice. Later on, he understood she had an excessive fear of conflicts. The atmosphere that had formed his pacific and soft ways was pietistic and overly friendly, but not very personal.

Another homosexual man had been reared by a single mother who hated anything that in her eyes was "aggressive". Thus she allowed him no "aggressive" toys, such as soldiers, army jeeps, or tanks; emphasized the physical and moral dangers that surrounded him; and had a somewhat hysterical ideal of nonviolent religious piety. That the son of this poor worrying woman became overly sensitive, dependent, fearful, and slightly hysterical himself is small wonder. He was incapacitated in his contact with boys and could only get along with one or two shy comrades, outsiders like himself. Let us anticipate our analysis of the homosexual wish by remarking that he became attracted to the "dangerous but exciting world" of the soldiers whom he often saw marching out of a nearby barracks. Those were strong men who lived in an unknown, fascinating world. That they intrigued him is, by the way, proof of his essentially normal manly instincts. Every boy wants to be a man, every girl wants to be a woman, and it is precisely when they feel incapacitated in that important field of life that they start idolizing others' masculinity and femininity.

To be clear, one must distinguish two separate steps in the development of homosexual feelings. The first is a "cross-gender" habit formation in interests and behavior, the second a masculinity/femininity inferiority complex (or gender inferiority complex) that may, but need not necessarily, arise on the basis of these habits. After all, there are effeminate boys and tomboyish girls who never become homosexually interested.

Further, the masculinity/femininity inferiority complex is usually not definitively formed until preadolescence or adolescence. A child may possess cross-gender qualities even at primary-school age, and a homosexual might retrospectively interpret that as proof that he had always been a homosexual, but that impression is wrong. Not until the self-perception of being inadequate as a man or woman—as a boy or girl—has taken firm root and is accompanied by self-dramatization (see below) and homoerotic fantasies can and should we speak of "homosexuality". In adolescence the die is cast, rarely before. Adolescence shows in many the famous "crack" or "bend" in the "curve of life" that was so familiar to an older psychology of mental development. Before adolescence, as we can learn from many homosexuals, life may have been uncomplicated and happy. Then came the clouds that have long darkened their inner firmament.

Prehomosexual boys are not typically boyish in that they are often "overdomesticated", soft, undaring, weak, while prehomosexual girls are sometimes rather aggressive, domineering, too "wild", or independent. When such children reach adolescence, these traits, for the most part stemming from the role they were educated in (e.g., "she looks like a boy"), subsequently, through these teenagers' comparing themselves with others of the same sex, help to shape their self-perception of gender inferiority. Even as the unmanly-feeling boy does not identify with his maleness, the unfeminine-feeling girl does not dare to identify with her feminine nature. One *avoids* what one feels inferior about. However, a preadolescent girl who dislikes playing with dolls or in general shuns feminine roles cannot be said to have a lesbian disposition already. Those who want to persuade youngsters that their homosexual fate is already sealed cause grave mental harm and commit grave injustice!

To complete the picture of predisposing factors for a gender inferiority complex, self-comparison with same-sex siblings may play an important role. In such cases, the boy was the "girl" among his brothers, and the girl was the "least girlish" among her sisters. Furthermore, seeing oneself as physically ugly is remarkably frequent. This category includes a boy's feeling that his face is too fine or girlish, or that he is sickly, handicapped, and so on, as well as a girl's feeling that her figure is unfeminine, that she is clumsy or not graceful in her movements, and the like.

Self-Dramatization and the Formation of an Inferiority Complex

Homosexuality is not adequately explained by a disturbed or detached relationship with the same-sex parent, and/or an overattachment to the opposite-sex parent, no matter how frequently these are associated with it. For one thing, such relationships are often seen in pedophiliacs as well, and in other sexual neurotics (Mohr et al. 1964, 61, 140). Moreover, there are normal heterosexuals with similar parent–child interactions. Secondly, as remarked above, neither do cross-gender behavior and interests necessarily lead to homosexuality.

Even a gender inferiority complex, however, may take various forms, and erotic fantasies flowing from it may not only be directed to young or more mature adults of the same sex, but also to children of the same sex (homosexual pedophilia), or possibly to persons of the opposite sex. The woman-chaser, for instance, often suffers from a variant of the masculinity inferiority complex. The decisive factor for homosexuality is the *fantasy*. And fantasy is shaped by self-image, the view of others—with regard to one's gender qualities—and chance events, such as determinative social contacts and experiences in puberty. The gender inferiority complex is the stepping-stone to a variety of frustration-borne sexual fantasies.

Feeling less masculine or feminine as compared to same-sex peers is tantamount to the feeling of *not belonging*. Many prehomosexual boys had the feeling of "not belonging" with their fathers, brothers, or other boys, and prelesbian girls with their mothers, sisters, or other girls. To illustrate the importance of "belonging" for gender identity and gender-conforming behavior, an observation by Green (1987) may serve. Of a pair of identical twin brothers, one became homosexual, the other heterosexual; the heterosexual was the one who bore his father's name.

"Not belonging", inferiority feelings, and loneliness interconnect. Now the question is, how do these feelings lead to homosexual desires? To see through this, the notion of "inferiority complex" must be clarified.

The child and the adolescent automatically react to feelings of inferiority and "not belonging" with *self-pity* or *self-dramatization*. They inwardly perceive themselves as pathetic, pitiable, poor creatures. The word "self-dramatization" is correct, for it describes the child's tendency to view himself as the tragic center of the world. "Nobody understands me"; "nobody loves me"; "everybody is against me"; "my life is all misery"—the young ego does not and for the most part cannot accept his sorrow, much less perceive its relativity or view it as something that will pass. The self-pity reaction is very strong, and it is easy to give way to it. For self-pity, to a degree, has a comforting effect, as does the pity one receives from other people in times of grief. Self-pity provides warmth; it consoles because there is something sweet in it. *Est quaedam flere voluptus*, there is a certain lust in crying, according to the ancient poet Ovid (*Tristia*). The child or adolescent who feels himself to be a "poor me" can become attached to this attitude, especially when he withdraws into himself and has no one to help him work through his problems with understanding, encouragement, and firmness. Self-dramatization is particularly typical in adolescence, when the young person easily feels a hero, special, unique, even in his sufferings. If the attachment to self-pity remains, then the complex proper, that is, the inferiority complex, comes into existence. In the mind, the habit of feeling like a "poor inferior me" is fixated. It is this "poor me" within who feels unmasculine, unfeminine, alone, and "not belonging" to the peer group.

Initially, self-pity works like good medicine. Rather soon, however, it works more like a drug that enslaves. At that point, it has become—unconsciously—a habit of self-comforting, of concentrated self-love. The emotional life has become *neurotic* essentially: addicted to self-pity. With the child's or adolescent's instinctive, strong egocenteredness this proceeds automatically, unless there are affectionate and strengthening interventions from the outside world. The ego will forever remain the hurt, poor one who pities himself; it remains the same child-ego. All views, efforts, and desires of the "child of old" have been preserved in this "poor me".

The "complex" is therefore fed by a lasting self-pity, by an *inner complaining about oneself*. Without this infantile (adolescent) self-pity, there is no complex. Inferiority feelings can exist temporarily, but if enduring self-pity takes root, they stay alive, often as fresh and strong when the person is fifty years old as when he was fifteen. "Complex" means that the

inferiority feelings have become autonomous, recurring, always active, though more intense at some times than at others. Psychologically, the person in part remains the child or
adolescent he was and no longer matures, or hardly, in the
area where the inferiority feelings reign. In homosexuals, this
is the area of self-image in terms of gender characteristics
and gender-related behavior.

As bearers of an inferiority complex, homosexuals are unconsciously self-pitying "adolescents". Complaining about
their psychical or physical condition, about being wrongly
treated by others, about their life, fate, and environment, is
typical with many of them, as well as with those who play
the role of being always happy. They are as a rule not aware
of their self-pity addiction. They see their complaints as
justified, not as coming from a *need* to complain and to feel
sorry for themselves. This need for misery and self-torment is
peculiar. Psychologically, it is a so-called *quasi-need* ("*Quasi-
Bedürfnis*"), an attachment to the pleasure of complaining
and self-pity, to playing the part of the tragic one.

Acquiring insight into the central neurotic drive of complaining and inner self-pity is sometimes difficult for therapists and others seeking to help homosexual persons. More
often than not, those who have heard about the self-pity concept think it a little far-fetched to assume that unconscious
infantile self-pity could be that basic to homosexuality. What
is generally remembered and agreed on concerning this explanation is the notion of "feelings of inferiority", not that
of "self-pity". The perception of the paramount role of infantile self-pity in neurosis and homosexuality is indeed new;
perhaps strange at first glance, but if thought over and
checked against personal observations it proves extremely en-
lightening.

3

HOMOSEXUAL DRIVES

The "Search for Love and Affection"

"Male affect starvation", Green (1987, 377) believes, "may motivate the later search for love and affection from males." Many modern homosexuality investigators have made this point. It is true provided one takes the masculinity inferiority complex with its self-pity into account. The boy may indeed have painfully missed the esteem and interest of his father, in other cases of his brother(s), or of his male peers, which made him feel inferior to other males. The ensuing urge for love is in fact the urge to belong to the men's world, to receive the recognition and friendship of those to whom he feels inferior.

At this point, we must avoid a common misunderstanding. There is a popular idea that people who did not receive (enough) love in childhood and who were psychologically affected by it will be cured if they now receive the lacking quantity of affection. Several therapeutic approaches have been based on this premise. But it is not that simple. First, it is not the objective lack of love that counts so much as the child's perception of it—and that by definition remains subjective. Children may misinterpret their parents' behavior and, with their tendency to dramatize themselves, may imagine they are not wanted, that their parents are terrible, and so on. Beware of taking the adolescent's view of his parents' treatment of him as an objective report!

Moreover, the "void of love" is not filled simply by pouring love into it. To be sure, that would be the solution the adolescent who feels lonely or inferior himself seeks and believes in. "If I receive the love I missed so much, I shall be happy", he imagines. But in accepting this theory one overlooks an essential psychological fact: the existence of the attachment to self-pity. Before the young person has become wont to experience himself as pitiable, affection indeed can help overcome his frustration. But once the "poor me" attitude has taken root, his love-seeking is no longer a functional, remedial drive, objectively aimed at reparation. It has become part of his self-dramatizing attitude: "I shall never get the love I want!" It is *insatiable longing*, never to be fulfilled. The search for same-sex love of the homosexual is a yearning that will not stop so long as the "poor me" attitude from which it flows remains alive. It was Oscar Wilde who complained, "I have always sought love and all I could find were lovers." The mother of a lesbian daughter who committed suicide observed: "All her life, Helen was looking for love", but of course she never found it (Hanson 1965, 189). Why not? Because she was addicted to her adolescent self-pity about *not being loved* by other women. Put otherwise, she was a "tragic adolescent". Homosexual love stories are dramas, not only frequently, but by their essence. The more lovers, the less the sufferer will be satisfied.

This mechanism of *pseudo-reparation* operates likewise in other affection-seeking people, and many neurotics recognize it in themselves. For example, a young woman had a series of male lovers, all of whom were comforting father figures to her. She felt badly treated by each of them in his turn, for she constantly pitied herself about not being loved (her relationship with father had been the starting point of her complex). How can affection cure one who is obsessed with the tragic idea of being "the rejected one"?

Seeking love as a means of comforting one's hurts may be passive and ego-centered. The other person is there only to love the "poor me". This is begging for love, not really mature *loving*. A homosexual may feel that he is the affectionate, loving, and protecting one, but in effect this is a game to attract the other to himself. It is all embedded in sentimentality and is profoundly narcissistic.

Homosexual "Love"

"Love" here must be put in quotation marks. For this is not real love such as male–female love (in its ideal state) may be or such as the love of normal friendships. What it is indeed is an adolescent sentimentality—puppy love—and erotic craving.

This blunt description may be taken by some as scandalous; looking at it this way may hurt the sensitive, but it is the truth. Fortunately, being confronted with this unflattering mirror can be salutary. One young homosexual man, for instance, acknowledged his masculinity inferiority complex, finding that insight to be a real help. But when it came to his romantic affairs, he was not at all certain that he could live without the "love" he sometimes encountered, which made life valuable. It might not be the ideal variant of love, but. . . . I explained that his love was pure childishness, *selfish self-pampering* and, therefore, imaginary. He was hurt, the more so because he was rather arrogant and presumptuous. However, after some months he phoned to tell me that though at first he had been furious, now he had "swallowed" it, and the effect was all right. He felt relieved, and several weeks had passed since he had inwardly distanced himself from seeking these egocentric contacts.

A middle-aged Dutch homosexual man told about his lonely childhood, when he had no friends and was an outcast among the boys because his father had been a member of the Nazi party. (I have seen many cases of homosexuality in children of these "traitors" in the last War.) Then he met a sensitive, understanding young priest and fell in love with him. This love had been the most beautiful experience of his life: there was a near-perfect mutual understanding; it really was serene and happy, but, alas, could not last for some reason or other. Such stories are likely to convince the naïve or the well-intentioned who want to be "caring", who conclude: "Then homosexual love *sometimes does* exist!" And why not sanction beautiful love, even if it does not conform to our personal standards? But let us not be deceived as this man deceived himself. He was wallowing in sentimental pubertal fantasies about the ideal friend he had always yearned for. He felt the helpless, pitiable, yet, oh, so sensitive, victimized little boy who at last *was* cherished by an admired, idolized friend. He was fully selfishly motivated in the relationship; indeed, he gave money to his friend and did many things for him, but only to buy his love. His inner mind-set was unmanly, begging, slavish.

The self-pitying adolescent admires exactly those who possess—as he sees it, anyhow—the characteristics he is lacking. As a rule of thumb, the heart of a homosexual's inferiority complex may be deduced from the traits he or she most admires in others of the same sex. If Leonardo da Vinci sought uncivilized boys of the street, we have reason to suppose he viewed himself as overly well-behaved and well-bred. French novelist André Gide felt he was an inhibited Calvinist boy who could not make contacts with the more adventurous boys of his age, and from that frustration sprang his frenetic admiration of boyish "good-for-nothings" and his longing for playful, intimate friendships with them. The boy with the worrisome, nonaggressive mother started admiring "soldier types" because he felt quite the opposite. Most homosexual men feel attracted to "masculine" young men, athletic types, men who are cheerful and make friends easily. Their masculinity inferiority complex becomes more apparent by that—effeminate men are unattractive to most homosexual men. The stronger a woman's lesbian emotions are, the less feminine she usually feels, and the more she looks for feminine types. Both partners of a homosexual "couple" —at least initially—are attracted to traits of physique or behavior in the other with regard to maleness (femaleness) that they feel they themselves do not have. In other words, they view the other's masculinity or femininity as "better" than their own, although in fact both may be deficient in masculinity or femininity. It is the same as with other inferiority complexes: one looks up to other people who are thought to possess the capacity or trait with regard to which one feels inferior, even if this inferiority feeling is objectively not justified. Apart from that, the man most desired for his masculine qualities or the woman most desired for her femininity is hardly ever available for a homosexual man or a lesbian woman, because precisely these types are usually heterosexual.

The adolescent's fantasies are chiefly what determine his homosexual "choice" of ideal (insofar as that may be called a "choice"). As with the boy who lived in the neighborhood of military barracks and developed fantasies about military men, chance plays a role in shaping these ideal fantasies. A girl who felt humiliated because the boys at school ridiculed her for being rather fat and "backwoods" (she helped her father with the farmwork) started admiring a charming, delicate girl in the classroom with fair hair and in every way different from herself. This "fantasy girl" was the model for her later lesbian interests. It is true that she did not feel especially close to her mother, and this factor contributed to her insecurity, but her lesbian interests as such awoke only when she was confronted with that particular girl. And it may be doubted that the lesbian fantasies would have come into existence or taken root if she could have actually become friends with this girl; in reality, her dream friend showed no interest in her. Puberty is the phase when girls are inclined to *gush over* girls or female teachers they admire. In that sense, lesbianism is but a fixation of this adolescent "gushing-over".

For the adolescent who feels inferior, admiration of idealized same-sex types produces eroticization. For what is desired is a close, exclusive, affectionate intimacy, warmth for the poor desolate soul one is. In puberty, not only is it common to idealize a person or a type of person but also to experience diffuse erotic feelings in connection with such persons. The need to be affirmed by an idol whose body and appearance are so highly admired, sometimes with desperate jealousy, may become a desire to be caressed and cherished by him or her, leading to erotic reveries.

A boy who feels like a sissy may in his fantasy be aroused by what he in his immature view sees as masculine symbols: men in leather clothes, with mustaches, driving motorcycles, and so on. Many homosexuals have a sexuality centered on *fetishes*. They are obsessed with underwear, a large penis, and so on, all indications of their pubertal sexual life.

What about the theory that homosexuals seek their father (or mother, alternatively) in their partners? I believe this is only partly correct, namely, insofar as some long for a fatherly (or motherly) approach from their partner, when they subjectively experienced a lack of fatherly or motherly love and recognition. Even in these cases, however, the search is more for a same-sex *friend*. In the fantasies of many, the fatherly/

motherly element is certainly not of the same paramount importance as their childhood or adolescence traumatization related to their peer group.

Adolescent eroticization of same-sex idols is not extraordinary in itself. The relevant question is why it becomes overwhelming in some, blocking most, if not all, heterosexual interests. The answer, as we have seen, lies in the adolescent's deep feelings of inferiority in relation to his same-sex peers, his feelings of "not belonging", and his self-pity. There is a parallel phenomenon in heterosexuality: girls who most hysterically idolize male pop-stars are likely to be the ones who feel lonely and think they are unattractive to boys. For the homosexually inclined, the stronger the feeling of being *hopelessly* "different", the stronger the fascination with same-sex idols.

Homosexual Sex Addiction

The homosexual lives in a fantasy world, first and foremost with regard to his sexuality. The adolescent comforts himself with the lust of romantic daydreams. He comes to see such intimate contacts as the solution to his misery, as paradise itself. He craves them, and the longer he cherishes these fantasies in his inner isolation or practices masturbation with such imaginings, the more he becomes enslaved to them. It is comparable to the attachment to alcohol and its artificial dreams of happiness in neurotics or otherwise unhappy people: a gradual slide into an unreal world of wishful fantasizing.

Frequent masturbation reinforces these love fantasies. Many young homosexuals practice it in a nearly compulsive way. Acceptance of and contentment with real life, however, are diminished by this form of narcissism, so there is a downward spiral as in other addictions; sexual gratification is sought ever more. After some time, the yearning for erotic contacts, in fantasy or reality, overruns the mind: one becomes obsessed with it, one's whole life seems to revolve around it. There is a constant search for prospective same-sex partners, an anxious scrutinizing of every candidate one meets. If we look for still another comparable psychological addiction, it is like gold-fever, or the obsession with power or riches of certain neurotics.

The "irresistible" fascination of maleness or femaleness to homosexually inclined persons explains their resistance to giving up their lifestyle, and also, for that matter, their homosexual daydreams. On the one hand, they are not happy with it, on the other, there is a powerful inclination to cherish it secretly. To give up homosexual lust seems equal to them to doing away with what makes life most worthwhile. This was so even when social disapproval of homosexuality was more apparent and homosexual acts were punishable by law. At that time, many active homosexuals preferred the risk even of repeated conviction to breaking off their cruising habits, as was observed by Dutch psychiatrist Janssens at a congress on homosexuality in 1939. Inherent in such behavior is the homosexual's penchant for misery; in a rebellious way, he prefers the drama of being jailed to a normal life. He is the tragic sufferer; the danger of punishment perhaps enhances the thrill of seeking homosexual contacts. In our day, it is not unusual for homosexuals purposely to seek HIV-infected partners from the same craving for tragic self-destruction.

Underlying and feeding the sex-craving is self-pity, the attraction to the tragic drama of impossible love. Therefore, homosexuals do not so much seek the other *person* in their sexual encounters as the materialization of impossible wish fantasies. The real other person is not seen as he is, and to the degree that he is experienced more realistically, this neurotic attraction correspondingly fades away.

Some supplementary notes on homosexual sex and other addictions: As with an alcohol or drug addiction, the satisfaction of the homosexual sex addiction (whether within or without a homosexual liaison, or by means of masturbation) is purely ego-centered. It is not a sharing of love but, stripped of the game that may be played, in essence an impersonal event, like contacts with a prostitute. The more "experienced" homosexual often agrees with this analysis. Ego-centered lust fills no void, only deepens it.

Furthermore, it is well-known that alcohol and drug addicts have a tendency to lie about their behavior, to others and to themselves. Sex addicts, among them homosexuals, may do the same. The married homosexual often lies about his infidelity to his wife, the one living in a homosexual partnership to his partner, the homosexual who wants to overcome his seeking homosexual contacts to his therapist and to himself. Some tragic cases are known of well-intentioned homosexuals who proclaimed they had broken away from the homosexual scene (through religious conversion, for instance) but who slipped back to a self-tormenting double-life (including the usual lying). This is understandable because it is difficult to be really radical and resolute in the decision to cease satisfying this addiction. In their desperation at thus failing, these people subsequently let themselves go without restraint, in a free-fall that can cause their psychological or physical destruction, like Oscar Wilde after his conversion in jail. In an attempt to put the blame for their weakness on others and to discharge their conscience, they may now bitterly defend the normality of homosexuality and denounce therapists or Christian counselors whose opinions they previously shared and whose directives they had embraced.

4

THE NEUROTICISM OF
HOMOSEXUALITY

Homosexual Relationships

It needs no further proof; the AIDS epidemic has made it
sufficiently clear that the vast majority of active homosexuals
are promiscuous, and much more so than promiscuous heterosexuals. The fairy tale of faithful homosexual "unions"
(with its slogan, "What is the difference from heterosexual
marriage, apart from the sex of the partner?") is a propaganda
item, to win privileges from the law and acceptance within
Christian churches. Years ago, German sociologist and homosexual activist Martin Dannecker (1978) already openly ad-
mitted that "homosexuals have a different sexual nature", i.e.,
that partner variability is inherent to their sexuality. The
"faithful marriage" concept had had its use in the strategy for
getting social approval for homosexuality, but now it was
time to drop the smoke screen, he wrote. Perhaps it was a
little premature for such honesty, for the opportunistic marriage concept still serves emancipatory purposes, in the legalization of adoption by homosexual couples, for example. So
a veil of lies and a repression of unwelcome facts still cover
the issue of relationships. In the Germany of the sixties and
early seventies, the well-known homosexual psychiatrist
Hans Giese never failed at any public discussion or forum on
homosexuality to hammer home the notion of the "faithful
and enduring partnership" of which his life would be an

example. But when he killed himself after one of his failed love affairs, the incident was pretty well passed over in silence by the media, as it was not exactly in support of the fidelity theory. Similarly, self-dramatization characterized the artistic career of the Belgian "singing nun" (Soeur Sourier) in the sixties. Breaking away from her convent to start a lesbian relationship, she asserted the viability of this "love", which she claimed could be in harmony with religious life itself. After some years she and her lover were found dead, allegedly having committed suicide together (if this is the true version; in any case, the scene indicated a romanticized "dying for love").

Two emancipatory homosexuals, a psychologist and a psychiatrist, David McWhirter and Andrew Mattison (1984), studied 156 male couples, the most partner-stable segment of the homosexual population. They concluded: "Though most gay couples begin their relationship with an implicit or explicit commitment to sexual exclusivity, only seven couples in this study had been consistently sexually monogamous." That is 4 percent. But notice what is meant with "consistently sexually monogamous": these men *said* they had had no other partners for a period of *less than five years*. Notice the authors' distorted use of language: "commitment to sexual exclusivity" is morally neutral and, in fact, a poor substitute for "fidelity". As for the 4 percent, we may safely predict that, even if they did not lie, the consistency of their behavior ended sometime soon afterward. Because that is the fixed rule. Homosexual restlessness cannot be appeased, much less so by having one partner, because these persons are propelled by an insatiable pining for the *unattainable* fantasy figure. Essentially, the homosexual is a yearning child, not a satisfied one.

The term *neurotic* describes such relationships well. It suggests the ego-centeredness of the relationship; the *attention-seeking* instead of loving; the continuous tensions, generally stemming from the recurrent complaint, "You don't love me"; the jealousy, which so often suspects, "He (she) is more interested in someone else." *Neurotic*, in short, suggests all kinds of dramas and childish conflicts as well as the basic disinterestedness in the partner, notwithstanding the shallow pretensions of "love". Nowhere is there more self-deception in the homosexual than in his representation of himself as a lover. One partner is important to the other only insofar as he satisfies that other's needs. Real, unselfish love for a desired partner would, in fact, end up destroying homosexual "love"! Homosexual "unions" are *clinging* relationships of two essentially self-absorbed "poor me's".

Self-Destructive and Dysfunctional Tendencies

The underlying dissatisfaction in the homosexual lifestyle is apparent from the high suicide rate of "self-proclaimed" homosexuals. Time and again, the gay lobby has dramatized the "conflicts of conscience", the "psychic emergency situation" homosexuals would be thrown into by those who declare homosexuality immoral or neurotic. They can be driven to suicide. I know of a case of suicide that was imputed by militant Dutch homosexuals to the victim's alleged "conscience conflict" because of his homosexuality, and they made as much as possible of it in the media. The dramatic story had been brought into the world by a friend of the deceased, a homosexual who wanted to take revenge because he was hurt by an unfavorable statement on homosexuality by an influential priest. In fact, his unhappy friend had not been homosexual at all. Committed homosexuals, the ones who allegedly have overcome their "imposed" conscience conflicts, kill themselves much more often than heterosexuals of the same age. A study by Bell and Weinberg (1978) found that over 20 percent of a large group of homosexuals had attempted suicide, 52 to 88 percent of them for reasons other than being a homosexual. Homosexuals may seek or provoke situations in which they can experience themselves as tragic heroes. Their suicidal fantasies sometimes take the form of dramatic "protests" against others, the world, to show how they are mistreated, misunderstood. Unconsciously, they want to wallow in self-pity. This is what motivated the strange behavior of Tschaikovsky, who purposely drank dangerously contaminated water from the Neva River and fell fatally ill. Like those neurotic romantics of the past century who threw themselves from the Lorelei rock in the Rhine to be drowned, homosexuals in our day may expressly seek AIDS-infected partners to ensure a tragedy for themselves. One homosexual proudly asserted that he had consciously contracted AIDS in order to form a "solidarity" with several of his friends who had died of it. The secular "canonization" of homosexuals who have died of AIDS is apt to stimulate such self-inflicted martyrdom.

Sexual dysfunctions also point to neurotic dissatisfaction. Of the homosexual couples in the study of McWhirter and Mattison, 43 percent reported forms of impotence. Compulsive masturbation is another symptom of neurotic sex; of the same group, 60 percent were said to masturbate two to three times a week (despite their sexual relationships). Many sexual perversions, notably masochism and sadism, are practiced by homosexuals, and highly infantile sexuality is no exception (e.g., underwear fixation, urinary and fecal sex).

Remaining a Teenager: Infantilism

The homosexual's personality is *in part* that of a child (or an adolescent). This phenomenon is known as the "inner complaining child". Some have emotionally remained teenagers in nearly all areas of behavior; in most, the "child" alternates with the adult in them, depending on place and circumstances.

The ways of thinking, feeling, and behaving typical of an adolescent who feels inferior are observable in the adult homosexual. He remains—in part—the defenseless poor loner he was in puberty: the shy, nervous, clinging, "abandoned", socially "difficult" boy who feels rejected by his father and peers because of his ugliness (squint-eyed, harelipped, or small, for example, he sees himself as the opposite of manly beauty); the pampered, self-admiring boy; the effeminate, arrogant, vainglorious boy; or the obtrusive, demanding, yet cowardly boy; and so on. The total boyhood (or girlhood) personality is preserved. This explains behavioral traits like the childish talkativeness of some homosexual men, their habits of weakness, naïveté, the narcissistic way they take care of their bodies, their way of speaking, and so on. The lesbian may remain the easily hurt, rebellious girl; the tomboy; the bossy girl driven by imitated masculine self-assertion habits; or the eternally wronged, sulking girl whose mother "had no interest in her"; and so on. The adolescent explains the adult. And everything is still there: views of oneself, one's parents, and others.

As noted earlier, an especially common view of self is that of the wronged, rejected, "poor me". Homosexuals therefore are easily insulted; they "collect injustice", as psychiatrist Bergler has so well put it, and are liable to see themselves as victims. This explains the overt self-dramatization of the militants, who adroitly exploit their neurosis to gain public support. Attached to self-pity, they are inner (or manifest) complainers, often chronic complainers. Self-pity and *protest* are not far apart. A certain inner (or overt) rebelliousness and hostility to others who do them wrong and to "society" and a determinate cynicism, are typical of many homosexuals.

This bears directly on the homosexual's difficulty in loving. His complex directs his attention to himself; he seeks attention and love, recognition, and admiration for himself, like a child. His self-centeredness thwarts his capacity to love, to be really interested in others, to take responsibility for others, to give and to serve (some kinds of serving, in fact, are means of getting attention and approval). But "how . . . is it possible for the child to grow up if the child is not loved?" homosexual author Baldwin wonders (Siering 1988, 16). Yet stating the problem that way only confuses the issue. For while a boy who longed for his father's love might indeed have been healed had he encountered an affectionate father-substitute, his remaining immature, however, is the consequence of the self-comforting reactions to a perceived lack of love, not the consequence of a lack of love in itself. An adolescent who succeeded in accepting his sufferings, forgiving those who did him wrong—for the most part without being aware of it—would suffer without becoming attached to self-centered self-pity and protest, and, in that case, his sufferings would make him mature. As human nature is ego-centered, such an emotional development is not likely to take place spontaneously, but there are exceptions, notably when an emotionally troubled adolescent meets a parent-substitute who encourages him in this direction. The way Baldwin presents the impossibility for the unloved child to grow up—he seems, in fact, to describe his own case—is too fatalistic and overlooks the fact that even a child (and certainly a young adult) possesses a degree of freedom and can *learn to love.* Many neurotics cling to this self-dramatizing attitude of "never having been loved" and incessantly demand love and compensation from others—from their marriage partners, friends, children, from society. The situation of many neurotic criminals is analogous. They may have, in fact, suffered from from a lack of love at home, even from abandonment, injury; yet their impulses to revenge themselves, their lack of mercy on the world that has been hard on them are *egotistical* reactions to a lack of love. Being ego-centered, a young person is in danger of becoming a seemingly incorrigible self-seeker—and sometimes one who hates others—when he is the prey of his self-pity. Baldwin was correct only insofar as his homosexual feelings were concerned, for they did not amount to real loving, but narcissistic longing for warmth, and envy.

The "inner child" views not only members of his own sex through the glasses of his gender inferiority complex, but also the opposite sex. "Half of mankind—the female half—did not exist for me, until recently", a homosexual client once said. He had viewed women as caring mother figures, as married homosexuals sometimes do, or as rivals in his hunt for male affection. Being too close to a woman his age can be threatening to a male homosexual, because he feels like a little boy who is not up to the male role in relation to adult women. This is true apart from the sexual element in the male–female relationship. Lesbian women may view men as their rivals too: they may want a world without men; men make them feel insecure and take their prospective woman friends from them. Homosexuals often view marriage and the male–female relationship without understanding, with envy and sometimes even hatred, because the "role" of manliness or womanliness itself annoys them; this is, in short, the view of an outsider who feels inferior.

In social respects, homosexuals (especially male) are sometimes addicted to collecting sympathy. Some make a veritable cult of their many, shallow friendships and have developed a skill for charming other people. They appear "extroverted". They want to be the most adored, the most loved boy of the group: an overcompensatory habit. They seldom feel on an equal footing with others, however: either inferior or superior (overcompensation). Overcompensatory self-affirmation bears the mark of childish thinking and childish emotionality. A shocking example is the small, ugly, squint-eyed Dutch homosexual youngster who, feeling unrecognized by his more handsome and more well-to-do peers, set out to realize his fantasy world of money, celebrity, and luxury (Korver and Govaars 1988, 13). He proved himself by acquiring impressive wealth when he was only in his early twenties; he gave tremendous parties in his Hollywood palace, inviting jet-set celebrities and spending a fortune on them—in fact, he bought their adoration and attention. He was the big star, handsomely dressed and made-up, surrounded by others. And he could have his lovers. But everything of his fantasy-world-become-reality in fact was a lie—his "friendships", the "adoration", his "beauty", and "social achievements". One who thinks about this kind of life can see how *unreal* it is. His fortune was built on drug trafficking and clever intriguing and cheating. His attitudes bordered on the psychopathic: he was indifferent to the fate of others, of his victims, and "stuck his tongue out" at society in vainglorious enjoyment of his sweet revenge. Never mind that he died of AIDS at age thirty-five, for, as he boasted not long before his death, *he* had had such a "rich" life. The psychologist can see the "child" in this mentality, the frustrated "child" who was the poor, ugly outsider craving for riches and friends; a child grown wicked, yet still unable to establish mature human bonds, miserably buying his friendships. His subversive mentality toward society flowed from his feeling of rejection: "I am not obligated to them!"

Subversiveness is not rare in homosexuals, as it is the hostility coming from the complex of "not belonging". For that reason, avowed homosexuals may be unreliable elements in any group or organization. The "inner child" within them continues to feel like the rejected one and cherishes rancorous reactions. There is an overcompensatory wish in many homosexual men and women to create a fantasy world "superior" to the ordinary, more "chic", snobbish, full of "thrill" and "adventure", of "curiosity" and expectation, of special encounters and friendships, but in fact full of irresponsible behavior and superficial contacts: adolescent thinking.

The emotional ties of persons with a homosexual complex to their parents remain as they were in childhood and adolescence: dependence on the mother, aversion, contempt, fear or indifference toward the father in the male; often ambivalent feelings as to the mother and (less often) emotional dependence on the father in the female. Such emotional immaturity is further reflected in the fact that not a few homosexuals are not deeply interested in children, in spite of outer appearances, as they are too self-absorbed and want all attention for themselves, as real children do.

For example, a homosexual man who, together with his friend, had adopted a daughter, later confessed that they had done it in order to show off, "as if she was a trendy pet dog; everybody looked at us when we, as ostentatious homosexuals, entered a room with her." Lesbian pairs who want to have a child have similar selfish aims. They "play the family", defying the real family, out of an insolent, provocative mindset. In some cases, they half-consciously want to play out lesbian practices with an adopted girl. The state that legalizes these unnatural situations is guilty of subtle, but grave, child abuse. In this field, the public is lied to, as it is with other homosexuality-related subjects, by social reformers who try to impose their sick ideas of the "family", including the homosexual family. To further the legalization of adoption by homosexual "parents", they quote studies that "prove" that children brought up by homosexuals are psychologically healthy. These "studies" are not worth the paper they are written on; they are pseudoscientific lies. Anyone who has more intimate information about a child thus "parented", and of his subsequent development, knows how bizarre and sad his situation has been. (On the manipulation of studies of homosexual parenting, see Cameron 1994.)

To summarize: ego-centered thinking and feeling—the chief characteristics of the psyche of the child and the adolescent—childishness and sometimes downright egotism pervade the child/adolescent personality of the adult with a homosexual complex. *His unconscious pity for himself, his viewing and treating himself as pitiable, as well as his "compensative" drives of attention-seeking, craving erotic contacts, and other ways of comforting and pampering himself are clearly infantile, i.e., ego centered.* Incidentally, "the child" is often intuitively perceived by others, who may take on a protective attitude toward a homosexual family member, friend, or colleague, treating him in fact as a "special", vulnerable child.

Doubtless, infantility marks homosexual "unions" and relations. Like two clinging boys or two immature girls, these adolescent bosom-friendships are full of infantile jealousies, rows, mutual nagging, provoking and bullying, and the inevitable final drama. If they "play marriage", it is a childish imitation, ridiculous and pitiable at the same time. A homosexual Dutch author, Louis Couperus, living at the beginning of this century, described his preadolescent longing for friendship with a cheerful, strong, protective uncle of his: Couperus "would wish to be with uncle Frank always, forever! And in his childlike fantasy he imagined that he was married to his uncle" (van den Aardweg 1965). Normal marriage is for the child the exemplar model of togetherness of two people. The two pathetic lonely "inner children" within two homosexuals may in their fantasy imitate this relationship—as long as the game will last. It is the fantasy of "two babes in the wood", two apart from the world. A magazine once featured a picture of the "marriage" celebration of two Danish lesbians in a town hall. Of course, it was a pubertal show of provocation and self-affirmation, but the marriage-game was obvious too. One of the two women, bigger and heavier, wore a groomlike black garment, the other, smaller and more slender, bride's clothes. Childish travesty of male–female roles and "eternal faithfulness". The most insane part, however, is normal people acting as if they seriously endorse such a game. If they were honest with themselves, they would have to admit that their intelligence and emotions really regard it as a sick joke.

Neurotic from Discrimination?

"I have been 'different' since I was a young child." Many homosexuals, perhaps half, can recall such a feeling. They err, however, if they equate this feeling of being different with being homosexual. The error of interpreting their being different in childhood as the expression and proof of a homosexual nature supports the wish to rationalize the homosexual lifestyle, as is the case with the well-publicized work of homosexual psychoanalyst R. A. Isay (1989). In the first place, his theory of homosexuality is in fact hardly a theory. He does not answer the question about the causes(s), deeming it "unimportant", since "you cannot do anything about it" (Schnabel 1993, 3). Even if that were true, this logic would be entirely unscientific. Is the question of what causes cancer, or delinquency, or alcoholism unimportant because today we cannot cure many forms of these conditions? The author comes off as being embittered and cynical as a result of his failure in marriage and psychoanalytic treatment. He tried, but did not succeed, and then resorted to the familiar self-justifying strategy: calling it a crime to try to change homosexuals, who are victims of discrimination, their "nature" being a sacred fact about which no questions should be asked. Numerous disillusioned homosexuals have reacted the same way; the French precursor of the homosexual movement, André Gide, when he left his wife and gave way to his pedophile adventures, took this dramatic stance back in the twenties: Here I stand; I can't help the way I am. This is the self-pitying defense of the loser, the defeatist. Understandable, perhaps, but still it is self-deception. The capitulating person knows he has failed for lack of persistence and honesty. Isay, for example, had gradually slipped into a double life of secret homosexual cruising while at the same time being the respectable family father and doctor. He was not unlike certain "ex-gays" who expect to get rid of their homosexuality by converting to Christianity, but cannot maintain their premature conviction of being "liberated" and eventually lose all hope. They have, moreover, a "guilty conscience". Their explanations are inspired not by logic, but by self-defense.

As a psychiatrist, Isay cannot deny the many "pathological and perverted" traits to be found in homosexuals (Schnabel 1993, 3), but he chooses to explain them as effects of the homosexual's lifelong rejection: by his father, his peers, society. If he is neurotic, then it is as a consequence of discrimination. This idea is not very original; homosexual clients who admit their neurotic emotionality but shrink from shedding critical light on their sexuality invariably resort to it. However, it is impossible to separate homosexual desire from neurosis. I have heard more than once from an applicant for therapy: "I want to get rid of my neurosis. It disturbs my homosexual liaisons. I want to have satisfactory sexual relations, but I do not want to change my homosexuality." How can one answer such a request? "If we work at your neurotic emotions and inferiority complex, your homosexual feelings will automatically be affected. Because they are manifestations of your neurosis." And so it is. The less depressed, the more stable emotionally, the less egocentric the homosexual person becomes, the less homosexually inclined he will feel.

On the surface, Isay's—and other homosexuals'—defensive theory may sound plausible; however, the more one confronts it with the psychological facts, the less it holds up. Assuming a child's "homosexual nature" was some mysterious given from birth on or originated soon afterward, would the vast majority of fathers automatically "reject" such a boy? Is it an iron rule that fathers are so cruel when they feel their sons are "different" in some diffuse way (their rejection taking place before anyone could be aware that this "difference" was a homosexual "nature")? For instance, do fathers as a rule reject sons with defects? No, of course not. Had the small boy this different "nature", then possibly a certain type of father would react with rejection, but certainly many more would instead respond with protection and help.

There is more. It is not among the great insights of child psychology to suppose that little boys start off with a tendency to be erotically infatuated with their father (which would flow from their homosexual nature, according to Isay). This view distorts reality. Many prehomosexual boys longed for personal warmth from their father, a hug, recognition, nothing erotic at all. Is that incomprehensible, when they were or felt "rejected"? What else would we expect, that the boy would be perfectly content with his father's attitude?

And then this feeling of being "different". There is no need for a mythical homosexual "nature" to explain it. A boy with feminine habits, who clings to his mother, was overprotected, or had no father or other manly influence in his tender childhood, *naturally* would feel "different" when confronted with other boys who had been able to develop their boyish inclinations and interests. On the other hand, feeling different is not, as Isay seems to imply, the dubious privilege of prehomosexuals. The majority of nonhomosexual neurotics experienced it in their youth as well; in other words, there is no reason whatsoever to see a homosexual disposition in it.

Isay's theory suffers from still other incongruities. Quite a few homosexuals did not have any feeling of "being different" *until* adolescence. They felt "one of the gang" in childhood but, due to migration, a change of schools, or other factors, developed a sense of isolation because they could not adapt to the others in their new environment, who were different socially, economically, or otherwise.

Finally, if one believes in the existence of a homosexual nature, then one must likewise believe in a pedophile nature, in fetishist, sadomasochistic, zoophile, transvestite natures, and others. There would be the specific "nature" of the exhibitionist who is sexually aroused by showing his penis to women who pass by his window. And the Dutch man recently arrested after having given in for eight years to an "irresistible" urge to watch women in the washroom could boast a voyeuristic "nature"! Then the young woman who had felt unwanted by her father and insatiably chased men ten years older than herself has a nymphomaniac "nature" that differs from the normal heterosexual nature, and her father-frustration was simply coincidental.

The homosexual author Isay depicts himself as the victim of a mysterious, dark fate; a view that is, in effect, pubertal self-tragedization. Considerably less flattering for the ego is the view that homosexuality is an attachment to immature emotionality! If Isay's theory of a homosexual "nature" were true, would then the homosexual's psychological immaturity, his remaining a "child", and his excessive preoccupation with himself be part of his, by principle irreducible and inexplicable, "nature"?

Neurotic by discrimination? A large number of homosexually inclined persons affirm they never suffered much from social discrimination, but much more from their own insight that they were not able to function normally. Immediately emancipatory homosexuals will react: "Yes, but this suffering is an internalization of social discrimination. They would not have suffered if society regarded homosexuality as normal." That is a cheap theory. Only those who repress spasmodically, who do not want to see, the self-evident biological unnaturalness of homosexuality and other sexual disturbances will buy that.

Otherwise, the order of events is not such that a child first realizes "I am a homosexual" and *subsequently* is neuroticized by others, or himself, because of it. A correct description of the psycho-history of homosexuals is that they first experienced the feelings of "not belonging", being inferior to the peer group, lonely, not being loved by a parent, and so on; and it is obvious that this is why they felt depressed and were neuroticized. The homosexual longing presented itself *after* and *as a consequence of* these experiences of rejection, not before.

Nonneurotic Homosexuals?

Do they exist? One would expect so, if social discrimination were the cause of the undeniably high frequency of neurotic emotional, sexual, and relational disturbances in homosexuals. But the nonneurotic homosexual is a fiction. That may be ascertained by observation as well as by the self-observation of homosexually inclined people. There is, moreover, a high correlation between homosexuality and

various psychoneuroses, such as obsessive-compulsive syn-
dromes and ruminations, phobias, psychosomatic problems,
neurotic depressions, and paranoid states.

As far as studies using psychological tests are concerned, all
groups of homosexually inclined people that have been examined with the best available tests[1] for neurosis or "neuroti-
cism" make high scores. It did not make a difference whether
or not those tested were socially adapted or "nonclinical",
they invariably scored as neurotics (for a review of the research, see van den Aardweg 1986).

Some people with this affliction may seem at first to be
nonneurotic. Sometimes it is said of a certain homosexual
person that he is always happy and contented, not problem-
atic. However, if one comes to know him more personally
and learns more about his private life and inner world, the
impression does not bear out. It is as with the alleged examples of "stable, happy, and faithful homosexual marriages":
on closer inspection the initial impression has to be corrected.

Normal in Other Cultures?

"Our Judeo-Christian tradition does not accept the homosexual 'variant', which in other cultures would be seen as
normal": here is another fairy tale. No culture or time has
considered homosexuality—understood as a stronger attraction to the same sex than to the opposite sex—normal.
Sexual practices among persons of the same sex may be accepted to a degree in some cultures, especially in relation to
initiation rites, but real homosexuality is always considered
abnormal.

[1] Warning: some tests are amateurishly presented as tests for neurosis,
though they definitely are not.

And it is often not as frequent in other cultures as in our own. How frequent is it with us, actually? Much less than is suggested by militant homosexuals and the media. One to two percent of the *adult* population at most, including bi-sexuals, has homosexual feelings. This percentage, which could be deduced from available samples (van den Aardweg 1986, 18), was recently confirmed by the Alan Guttmacher Institute (1993) for the U.S. In Great Britain, it appears to be 1.1 percent (Wellings et al. 1994; the best compilation of data on the incidence one can find is in Cameron 1993, 19).

In a small New Guinea tribe, the Sambia, no more than one of several thousand tribesmen could be found who was a homosexual; in fact, he was a pedophiliac (Stoller and Herdt 1985, 401). The man was described as abnormal not only in sexuality, but in behavior as well: he was "cold", "uncomfort-able in public" (indicating feelings of inferiority, insecurity), "secretive", "moody", "noted for his sarcasm". A neurotic picture, apparently that of the outsider who feels inferior and has taken a hostile attitude to the "others".

This man was "different" in that he avoided as much as possible the manly activities of hunting and fighting, while he preferred gardening, his mother's occupation. His social-psychological position gave clues to the origins of his sexual neurosis. He was the only and illegitimate son of a woman who had been deserted by her husband and was therefore despised by the whole tribe. It seems probable that the lonely and outcast woman had bound the boy very much to herself, so that he did not grow up as a boyish boy—not too different from those prehomosexual boys in our culture, who were only children and lived symbiotically with their mothers, in the absence of a father. The child was reared by a mother who was embittered toward all men, and thus, we may guess, not likely to make "a real man" of him. Social isolation and rejection characterized the childhood of this

boy—the inferior son of an abandoned woman. It is significant that he had had homosexual fantasies since preadolescence, in contrast with the other boys of his age. *Fantasies*
make for the crucial difference, not sexual practices in themselves. This is obvious here, for *all* Sambia boys were taught
to have sex with young men, playing at first the passive role,
and, grown older, contacting younger boys and playing the
active part. The rationale of these initiation practices is that
the adolescent will acquire the strength of the young men.
In their early twenties, they marry. Now, the remarkable
thing is that, as marriage approaches, the young men naturally turn to *heterosexual fantasies*, and after marriage there is
no homosexual desire, in spite of the former habit of passive
as well as active homosexuality. The exceptional homosexual
pedophiliac of the tribe studied by Stoller and Herdt had
apparently not been deeply emotionally involved when he,
too, had practiced sex for some time with young *men*, for his
erotic fantasies centered on *boys*. From this it must be in-
ferred that he had felt traumatically rejected by his boyhood
group and had felt different, mainly from other *boys*, the outsider.

The Sambia example makes it clear that homosexual practices must not be equaled to homosexual interests. "Real"
homosexuality is rather rare in most cultures. An educated
man from Kashmir once expressed to me his conviction that
homosexuality did not exist in his country, and I heard the
same from a priest who had worked for more than forty years
in northeast Brazil, he himself being a native of the region.
Perhaps, we might object, there are hidden cases. But that is
far from certain. One might as well suppose that the clear
distinction being made in those regions between boys and
girls and the unanimous treatment of a boy as a boy and a girl
as a girl, with the accompanying respect, are highly preven-
tive. Boys are encouraged to feel like boys, and girls like girls.

Seduction

The Sambia study may help in understanding the contribution of seduction to the development of homosexuality. Seduction cannot be regarded a decisive causative factor in children and adolescents with normal self-confidence in the area of gender. But it is perhaps more important than has been thought for several decades. An English study found that, although 35 percent of questioned boys and 9 percent of girls reported having experienced a homosexual seduction attempt, only 2 percent of these boys and 1 percent of these girls had responded. But then, we can look at it from a different angle. It is not unrealistic to assume that seduction *can* do harm when the young person is already developing a gender inferiority complex, or when his pubertal fantasies have begun to be focused on same-sex objects. Seduction may, in other words, strengthen an ongoing homosexual development, and sometimes even enkindle homosexual desires in youngsters who are insecure in their gender. I have been told this a couple of times by homosexual men. A typical story runs this way: "There was a homosexual man who was kind to me and gave me affection. He seduced me, and at first I loathed it. But some time later I started fantasizing about having sexual contact with another young man whom I admired and whose friendship I sought." Seduction therefore is not so innocent as some want us to believe (such an idea is propaganda for the normalization of pedophilia and for child adoption by homosexuals). Likewise a "sexual atmosphere" in the home—pornography, homosexual videos and movies—can also reinforce still uncertain homosexual interests. Some homosexuals would in all likelihood have been heterosexual if homosexual fantasy had not been aroused in them during the critical period of their emotionally unstable adolescence. They would probably have quietly outgrown their pubertal, and still at most *superficially* erotic, admiration of same-sex friends and idols. In some girls, heterosexual seduction facilitated, or enhanced, already existing homosexual interests. It cannot, however, be considered an isolated cause; we must not lose sight of the connection with previously developing feelings of being unwomanly.

5

THE QUESTION OF MORALITY

Homosexuality and Conscience

Conscience is a much neglected subject in modern psychology and psychiatry. Its morally neutral substitute, the so-called Freudian superego, cannot account for the psychological dynamics of man's *authentic moral conscience*. The superego is defined as the sum of all learned rules of behavior. "Good" and "bad" behavior do not depend on moral absolutes, but on cultural, essentially arbitrary, codes. The philosophy behind this theory is that norms and values are relative and subjective: "Who am I to say what is good or not for you, what is normal and abnormal?"

But, in fact, everyone, including modern man, in one way or another, be it more clearly or more vaguely, "knows" of the existence of "eternal" moral laws, as they were called even by the ancients, and directly and spontaneously recognizes stealing, lying, cheating, infidelity, murder, rape, and so on, as *intrinsically evil* (evil in themselves) and generosity, courage, honesty, and faithfulness as *intrinsically good*, beautiful. While immorality and morality are most evident in the behavior of others (Wilson 1993, 11),[1] we still perceive these

[1] An illustration of the psychological fact that one's own sexual desires are not so clearly recognizable as immoral as are those of others is the moral disgust of many homosexuals to pedophile sexuality. In an interview, an

qualities in our own behavior as well. There is an inner perception of the intrinsic wrongfulness of certain deeds and plans, however much the ego is inclined to repress that perception so as not to have to give up those deeds and plans. This inner, moral judgment of self is the working of the authentic conscience. Although it is true that some manifestations of moral self-criticism are neurotic and that the perceptions of conscience can be distorted, for the most part, human conscience points to objective moral realities, which are more than mere "cultural prejudices". It would take us too far to corroborate this view with psychological data and facts. For the critical observer, however, the evidence for the "authentic conscience" is everywhere.

These notes are not superfluous, because conscience is a psychic factor that is easily neglected in the discussion of a theme like homosexuality. For instance, we cannot overlook the phenomenon of the *repression of conscience*, which, according to Kierkegaard, is much more important than the repression of sexuality. Repression of conscience is never perfect, not even in the so-called psychopath. In the depth of the heart, there remains a certain awareness of *guilt*, or, in the Christian term, of one's *sinfulness*.

Knowledge of the authentic conscience and its repression is extremely important for any kind of "psychotherapy". For conscience is always a participant in motivation and behavior.

Amsterdam homosexual porno-magnate gave vent to his indignation over the pedophile activities of a colleague of his; such actions were "immoral": "sex with such young kids!" And he expressed his hope that the perpetrator would be convicted and get a good spanking (*De Telegraaf* 1993, 19). Automatically, the word comes to mind: "this is *dirty*", using innocent children and adolescents for one's perverted lust. This man proved his capacity for normal moral reactions to the behavior of other people; but then, he was value-blind when it came to his own attempts to seduce young and old to a variety of homosexual practices and to his earning so much money thereby—exactly as blind as the pedophiliac was to *his* immorality.

Therapists who have no eye for it cannot really understand what is going on in the inner life of many clients and run the risk of misinterpreting important aspects of their lives in a detrimental way. Not making use of the light of the client's conscience, however dim it be, means that we will fail to find the best means, the right strategies. No modern behavior scientist has underlined the central function of the authentic conscience—rather than its Freudian ersatz—in the personality, even in seriously disturbed mental patients, more emphatically than the famous French psychiatrist Henry Baruk (1979).

For many in our day, it is more difficult, however, to persuade themselves that, in addition to the existence of general moral absolutes, there must also be universal moral values in matters of sexuality. But despite the reigning liberal sexual ethics, many kinds of sexual behavior and desires are still generally called "dirty" or "unsavory"; in other words, people's *feelings* with respect to immoral sex have not really changed (particularly when it concerns the behavior of *others*). Sexual lust sought exclusively for oneself, with or without the assistance of another person, particularly arouses feelings of aversion, even loathing, in other persons. Conversely, self-discipline in normal sexuality—*chastity* being the Christian term—is almost universally respected and honored.

That sexual perversions have always and everywhere been regarded immoral has to do with their unnaturalness and purposelessness, but also with their total self-centeredness. In the same way, uninhibited, gluttonous eating or drinking and greediness for possessions are felt by other persons, by those observing these behaviors, as disgusting. Homosexual behavior is thus one of the sexual behaviors that inspire abhorrence in other people. This is why homosexuals who advocate their lifestyle do not attract attention to their sexual practices, but instead concentrate on the representation of homosexual "love". And to counterattack the psychologically normal aversion to homosexual activities, they invented the idea of "homophobia", thus perverting what is normal into something abnormal. But many of them admit that they feel guilty about their behavior (a former lesbian, for instance, describes her "sense of sin" in Howard 1991), and not only those with a Christian upbringing. Many express their disgust with themselves after having homosexual contacts. Guilt symptoms are present even in those who proclaim that their contacts were nothing less than beautiful. Certain manifestations of unrest, tension, an incapacity for real gladness, an urge to accuse and provoke can be ascribed to the stirrings of a "guilty conscience". For sex addicts, it is indeed difficult to recognize a deeply underlying and hidden moral dissatisfaction with themselves. Sexual desire tends to cloud the usually weaker moral feelings, which, however, cannot be completely smothered.

Actually, then, the most definitive and best argument for a homosexual to utilize against indulging his fantasies is his own innermost feeling for what is pure and what is impure. But how does one bring that to clear consciousness? By sincerity to oneself and quiet reflection, by learning to listen to one's conscience, and learning *not* to listen to such inner arguments as: "Why not?" or "I can't let go of satisfying these urges" or "I have a right to follow my nature." Reserve some time, some weeks, for this process of learning-to-listen. Walk around for some time with the honest question: How do I myself, if I carefully and without prejudice open myself to my deepest stirrings, feel about behaving in a homosexual manner? and about abstaining from it? It is only the sincere and courageous ear that will hear the answer, that becomes aware of the directives of conscience.

Religion and Homosexuality

A young, homosexually inclined Christian told me he had studied the Bible and found reasons to reconcile his conscience with his homosexual relationship of that moment, provided he remained faithful. Predictably, after some time he dropped that pretension, but he continued on his course, and his Christianity withered. That is the history of many young persons who try to reconcile the irreconcilable. If they convince themselves that homosexuality is morally good and beautiful, they either lose their faith or invent one of their own, which sanctions their desires. Of the last possibility, examples abound as well as of the first. A well-known homosexual Dutch actor from a Catholic background, for instance, presently plays the role of self-appointed priest, "blessing" young couples at marriage celebrations (not excluding homosexual "couples", of course) and "ministering" at funerals.

This brings up a topic of current interest: Why are so many Protestant and Catholic homosexuals, male and female alike, interested in theology, and why do they not infrequently want to be ministers or priests? Part of the answer lies in their infantile need for sympathy and contact. They view church professions as soft and sentimentally "caring" and imagine themselves in them as being honored and revered, elevated above common human beings. They see the Church as a noncompetitive, friendly world where they may enjoy high status and be protected at the same time. For male homosexuals, there is the additional incentive of a rather closed men's community where they need not prove themselves as men; women with lesbian feelings, on their part, may feel drawn to an exclusive women's community, like a convent. Unctuous ways, which they associate with "pastoral" manners and ways, moreover, appeal to some, being in line with their overfriendly, soft manners. And in the Catholic and Russian Orthodox Churches, there is the attraction of the garments and the aesthetic rituals, which male homosexuals may, in their childish perception, experience as feminine and which enable a narcissistic showing off, comparable to the exhibitionistic joys of homosexual ballet dancers.

Remarkably, lesbian women may also feel attracted to the role of vicar and priest. In their case too the attractive element for those who feel they don't belong is the social recognition as well as the enjoyment of being able to dominate others. It is interesting that the attraction of homosexuals to priestly functions is not restricted to modern Christianity; in several primitive societies, as in antiquity, homosexuals have fulfilled the priestly role.

These interests stem for the most part, then, from an infantile, self-centered imagination and have precious little to do with the objective contents of Christian belief. What some homosexuals thus see as their "calling" to the priesthood is an attraction to an emotionally rewarding, but self-centered, way of life. These are self-imagined or "false" vocations. Needless to say, these ministers and priests are inclined to preach a soft, humanistic reinvention of traditional beliefs, especially of moral principles, and a distorted concept of "love". Moreover, they tend to create a homosexual subculture within their churches. There they undoubtedly pose a subtle threat for the orthodoxy and undermine church unity by their habit of forming subversive coteries that do not feel responsible to the official church community (the reader may recall the homosexual complex of "not belonging"). Otherwise, they generally lack the balance and the strength of character necessary for giving fatherly guidance.

Do real vocations never go along with homosexual interests? I do not dare to affirm that fully; perhaps I have seen a few exceptions in the course of the years. But, as a rule, a homosexual orientation, whether acted out or experienced only in the private emotional life, must certainly be regarded as a contraindication to the supernatural source of priestly interests.

PART TWO

PRACTICAL RULES FOR
(SELF-)THERAPY

6

THE ROLE OF THERAPY

Sobering Remarks on "Pyschotherapy"

If I make a correct estimate, "psychotherapy" has had its best years. The twentieth century has been the age of psychology and psychotherapy. Great expectations were aroused by these new sciences, which promised great discoveries in the human mind and new methods of behavior modification and of curing mental problems and diseases. It turned out otherwise, however. Most "discoveries", like many ideas from the Freudian and neo-Freudian schools, proved illusory—even if they still find their tenacious adherents. Psychotherapy fared no better. The boom in psychotherapies (the 1980 *Psychotherapy Handbook* by Herink listed more than 250 of them) seems to have come to an end; and in spite of its social institutionalization, which has been hopelessly premature, the hope of the great returns of psychotherapy has dwindled. The first doubts concerned the illusions of psychoanalysis. Before World War II, such an experienced analyst as Wilhelm Stekel told his pupils that "if we do not make real new discoveries, psychoanalysis is doomed." In the sixties, confidence in psychological therapeutic methods was displaced by the seemingly more scientific "behavior therapies", but they too did not vindicate their pretensions. Nor did so many other new schools and "techniques" that presented themselves as breakthroughs, and often even as royal roads to cure and happiness. In fact, most of them consisted of warmed-up leftovers of older notions that were rephrased and commercialized.

What seem to remain, after so many beautiful theories and methods have gone up in smoke—a process that is still under way—are a few relatively simple ideas and general experiences. Not much, but still it is something. For the most part, we have returned to traditional psychological knowledge and wisdom, perhaps deepened here and there, but without the sensational developments found in physics or astronomy. Yes, it even becomes increasingly clear that we have to "rediscover" old truths that have been obscured by the semblance of superiority of the new psychologies and psychotherapies—for example, insights into the existence and workings of conscience, on the value of virtues such as courage, contentment, patience, altruism versus ego-centeredness, and the like. As for the effectiveness of psychotherapeutic methods, the situation can be compared to unlearning a dialect one has spoken since childhood—and this can be done, too—or to methods for quitting smoking: you can be successful, provided you fight the habit. I say "fighting" for no miracle cures can be expected. Likewise, there are no ways of overcoming the homosexual complex by remaining comfortably passive ("Bring me under hypnosis and I'll wake up a new man"). Methods or techniques are helpful, but their effectiveness depends greatly on realistic insight into one's character and motives and on a sincere and steadfast will.

"Psychotherapy", if it is sound, can offer valuable points of insight about the origins and structure of troublesome emotional and sexual habits, but not discoveries that will cause a change overnight. For instance, no psychotherapy can provide a sudden liberation, as is pretended by certain "schools", by unblocking repressed memories or emotions. There are no shortcuts through ingeniously devised learning techniques based on alleged new insights into the laws of learning, either. What is required is much common sense and quiet, daily perseverance.

The Need for a Therapist

What about the necessity for a therapist? Apart from extreme exceptions, the principle to remember is: One cannot go it alone. Normally, the person who tries to work himself through his neurotic complex badly needs another person to *guide* or *coach* him. In our culture, a psychotherapist is one who specializes in this work. Unfortunately, many psychotherapists are not qualified for helping homosexuals overcome their complex as they have hardly any idea of what this condition is about and share the prejudice that nothing can or should be done about it. So, for many who want to change but cannot find a professional helper, the "therapist" must be a person with a good dose of common sense and normal psychological insights, one who knows how to observe and has experience in guiding people. He should possess a good intelligence and be effective in establishing a rapport. Above all, he must have a balanced, normal personality and sound morals. He may be a pastor, minister, or priest, a physician, a teacher, a social worker—although these professions do not automatically guarantee therapeutic talents. I would advise the homosexually afflicted person to ask someone he senses has enough of the above qualities to guide him. Let the willing amateur therapist see himself as a helping older friend, a father, not having any scientific pretensions, but one who soberly uses his brains and normal human wisdom. He must learn something about the homosexual condition, no doubt, and I offer him this work to enhance his insight. It is not advisable, however, to read too many books on this subject, as much of the literature tends to confuse the reader.

The "client" needs a guide. He has to ventilate his emotions, express his thoughts, tell his life-story. He must discuss how his homosexuality came about, how his complex functions. He must be encouraged to fight in a regular, quiet, and sober way; he must also be checked in his fighting. Everyone who wants to play a musical instrument knows that it will not work without regular lessons. The teacher explains, corrects, stimulates; the pupil works from lesson to lesson. So it is with any form of psychotherapy.

Sometimes, "ex-homosexuals" help others to overcome their problem. They have the advantage of knowing the inner life and difficulties of the homosexual from firsthand experience. Moreover, if really completely changed, they incorporate for their friends the hopeful possibility of change. Yet I am not always enthusiastic about this undoubtedly well-meant solution to the therapeutic question. A neurosis like homosexuality may have been largely overcome, yet various related neurotic habits and mind-sets, apart from the danger of occasional relapses, may remain for a long time. Functioning as a therapist should in such cases not be attempted too soon; one must have lived for at least five years with a total inner change, including having heterosexual feelings, before taking up such a task. As a rule, however, the "real" heterosexual can best inspire heterosexuality in the homosexual client, and the one who has no problems with his masculine identity can best stimulate masculine self-confidence in one who lacks it. In addition, trying to "cure" others may unconsciously be a self-assertive means for one who is avoiding working seriously on himself. And sometimes, a subtle wish to continue contact with the homosexual "sphere of life" may mingle with the upright intention to help others who are in difficulties he knows so well himself.

I spoke of the fatherly male therapist or his lay stand-in. What about the female? For this kind of therapy with adults, I do not believe women are the best option, not even in cases of lesbian clients. Some understanding conversations and encouragement by female friends and guides may certainly be supportive; nonetheless, the long job (requiring years) of coaching and leading the homosexual with a consequent and firm hand requires a father figure. I do not see this as discriminatory toward women, because pedagogy and upbringing consist of two elements, the male and the female. The mother is the more personal, spontaneous, affective educator, the father more the leader, the coach, the teacher, the curb, and the authority. Women therapists are better suited for child therapy and female-adolescent therapy, men for the kind of *pedagogy* that requires male leadership qualities. Think of the fact of life that mothers generally have difficulties bringing up their adolescent and young adult sons (and not seldom, their daughters too!) when there is no father around with his manly authority.

7

KNOWING ONESELF

Working through Childhood and Adolescence

Self-knowledge is, first of all, *objective* knowledge of one's "character" or personality, i.e., one's motivations, attitudes, habits; it is the knowledge of ourselves *others* would have if they knew us well. It is much more than knowledge of our *subjective* emotional experiences. But for self-understanding one must also know one's psychological history and have a reasonably clear notion of how one's character and neurotic dynamics came about.

Very probably, the homosexually inclined reader has automatically referred to himself much of what was brought to the fore in the preceding chapters. The reader who wants to apply these ideas to himself—who wants to be his own therapist—would do well, however, to go over his psychological history more systematically. To this end, I present the following questionnaire.

The best method is to write down your answers, in order to make your ideas on yourself as clear and concrete as possible. Look at your answers again after about a fortnight and correct what you think needs to be amended. Often one discerns certain relationships better after having let the questions sink into one's mind for a while.

Anamnestic Questionnaire (Your Psychological History)

1. Describe your emotional relationship with your father while you were growing up. Which of the following characteristics apply to your relationship: familiarity, encouragement, identification, etc.; or distance, feelings of being criticized, feelings of lack of acceptance, fear, hatred, or contempt of him; a conscious longing for his sympathy and attention, etc.? Write down which characteristic(s) suit(s) you best, adding any characteristics that are missing from this short summary. A differentiation as to period of development may need to be made, for example: "Up to puberty (until about 12 to 14 years), our relationship was . . . ; afterward, however. . . ."

2. What did I think (especially in puberty/adolescence) my father thought of me? This inquires into the young person's view of his father's view of him. The answer may be, for instance: He found me uninteresting; he esteemed me less than my brothers (sisters); he admired me; he favored me, etc.

3. Describe your relationship with him now, and how you behave toward him. For instance, are you close, friendly, at ease, respectful, etc., or hostile, quarreling, tense, provoking, fearful, distant, cold, arrogant, rejective, fostering rivalry, etc.? Write down your own characteristic attitudes and behaviors toward your father as you usually display them.

4. Describe your feelings for your mother and your relationship with her during childhood and puberty (the answer may have to be divided). Was it familiar, warm, close, relaxed, etc., or constrained, fearful, distant, cool, etc.? Specify your answer, choosing those characteristics that you think are most typical in your case.

5. How do you think your mother regarded you (during childhood and adolescence)? What was her view of you? For instance, did she see you just "normally", as the boy or girl

you were, or did she regard you in some special way, as her intimate friend, her favorite, her ideal or model child, etc.?

6. Describe your current relationship with your mother (see question 3).

7. In what way were you reared by your father (or grandfather, stepfather)? For instance, according to a protective, encouraging, disciplining, free, trustful, confident "method"; with many worries and complaints; in a strict, over-disciplining, demanding, critical way; in a hard, or soft, indulgent, pampering, infantilizing, or babying way? Add any characteristic left out of this list that would better describe your case.

8. What methods did your mother use in bringing you up? (See question 7 for characteristics.)

9. How did your father regard and treat you as far as your sexual identity was concerned? With encouragement, appreciation, as a real boy or girl, or with little respect, with little appreciation, with criticism, contempt, etc.?

10. How did your mother regard and treat you with regard to your sexual identity? (See question 9.)

11. Where did you fall in birth order among your siblings (only child; first of _____ children, second of _____ children, last of _____ children, etc.)? In what way did this affect your psychological position and treatment within the family? For instance, an "afterthought" child may have been more protected or pampered; the only boy among several girls is likely to have had a different position and treatment as compared with the eldest of more boys, etc.

12. How did you see yourself compared to your same-sex siblings? As preferred by father or mother, as "better" in some capacity or character trait, or as less valuable?

13. How did you see your masculinity or femininity as compared with your same-sex siblings?

14. Did you have same-sex friends in childhood? What

was your position among your same-sex peers? For instance, were you one with many friends, popular, a leader, etc., or an outsider, a follower, etc.?

15. How about your same-sex friendships in puberty? (See question 14.)

16. Describe your contacts with the opposite sex in childhood and puberty, respectively (for instance, none, or associated exclusively with the opposite sex, etc.).

17. For men: Did you as a boy play with soldiers, war toys, etc.? For women: Did you play with dolls, stuffed animals?

18. For men: Were you interested in baseball or soccer? Furthermore, did you play with dolls? Were you interested in clothes? Specify.

For women: Were you interested in clothes and make-up? Furthermore, did you play boys' games by preference? Specify.

19. Were you either verbally or physically aggressive and self-affirming as an adolescent, moderately so, or just the opposite?

20. What were your principal hobbies and interests during adolescence?

22. How did you see your body (or parts of it), your physical appearance (for instance, as beautiful or ugly)? Specify as to what physical attributes distressed you (figure, nose, eyes, penis or breasts, height, fatness or thinness, etc.).

22. How did you see your body/physical appearance in terms of being male or female?

23. Did you have any physical handicap or illness?

24. How was your usual mood in childhood, and, secondly, in adolescence? Cheerful, sad, temperamental, or constant?

25. Did you go through any specific periods of inner desolation or depression in childhood or adolescence? If so, how old were you? And do you know why?

26. Did you have an inferiority complex as a child or as an adolescent? If so, in what specific areas did you feel inferior?

27. Can you describe what kind of a child/adolescent you were in terms of your behavior and tendencies during the period you felt your inferiority most acutely? For instance: "I was a loner, very independent of everyone, withdrawn, self-willed"; "I was shy, overcompliant, servile, lonely, yet angry inside"; "I was like a baby, easily brought to tears, yet pedantic"; "self-affirming, attention-seeking"; "I was always pleasing, smiling, and easy-going on the outside, but inwardly I was unhappy"; "I played the comedian"; "I was overly compliant", "a coward", "a leader", "domineering", etc. Try to remember the salient characteristics of your childhood or adolescent personality.

28. What other important things played a role in your childhood and/or adolescence?

As to the *psychosexual history*, the following questions will help to guide you:

29. At about what age did you feel your first infatuation with a person of the same sex?

30. What physical or personality type was he or she? Describe what attracted you most in him or her.

31. Approximately how old were you when you felt your first homo*sexual* inclination or fantasy? (The answer may be identical with that to question 29, but not necessarily so.)

32. What kind of persons usually arouse your sexual interest, in terms of age, physical or personality traits, behavior, or dress? Examples for men include: young men from 16 to 30 years, preadolescent boys, feminine types, masculine types, athletic types, motherly types, soldiers, slender types, blonde or dark-haired types, popular types, easy-going types, "rough" types, etc. For women: young girls, age _____;

middle-aged women with certain characteristics; women my age; etc.

33. If applicable, with what frequency did you practice masturbation in puberty? And thereafter?

34. Have you ever had spontaneous heterosexual fantasies, with or without masturbation?

35. Have you ever had erotic feelings toward or infatuations for someone of the opposite sex?

36. Are there any peculiarities in your sexual practices or fantasies (masochism, sadism, etc.)? Describe succinctly and soberly which fantasies or behaviors of others are exciting to you, for these may reveal something about the areas in which you feel inferior.

37. After having thought over and answered these questions, write a short life history containing the most important developments and inner events of your childhood and adolescence.

Knowledge of the Present Self

This part of self-insight is essential; insight into one's psycho-history, the subject of the previous section, is in fact useful only insofar as it promotes insight into the present self, that is, the present habits, emotions, and, most important of all, motives that are related to the homosexual complex. For effective (self-)treatment, it is essential that one comes to see oneself in an objective light, as another person who knows us well would see us. Indeed, observations by such others are often of great importance, especially when they come from persons who share our normal daily activities. They may open our eyes to habits or attitudes to which we are blind or which we would never admit. Here then is the first method of acquiring this self-insight: collect and carefully consider remarks made by others, including those whom you do not like.

The second method is *self-observation*. It primarily focuses on inner events—emotions, thoughts, fantasies, motives/drives—and secondarily on outward behavior. As to the latter, we can try to represent how we behaved, as if we were looking at ourselves, like a second ego, objectively, from a certain distance. Of course, inner self-perception and representation of our behavior through the eyes of an onlooker are interconnected processes.

Self-therapy, like standard psychotherapy, commences with an introductory period of self-observation, about one or two weeks. It is good practice to keep notes of these observations regularly (though not necessarily every day, only if there is something of importance to note), to write them down soberly, but straightforwardly. Use a special notebook for that purpose and make a habit of jotting down your observations, as well as questions or critical reflections. Writing increases the sharpness of observations and insights. Moreover, it enables one to study them some time later, which many experience as even more revealing than noting them at the moment of their occurrence (or soon afterward).

What should be recorded in the self-observation diary? Avoid keeping merely a *book of complaints*. People with neurotic emotionality tend to ventilate their frustrations and thereby to complain about themselves in such a self-observation diary. If, after some time, they recognize their self-complaining in re-reading their notes, then this is pure gain. They perhaps have unwittingly registered their self-pity truthfully at the time, so they can later make the discovery: "Oh, how I *did* feel sorry for myself!" The best policy, however, in writing down one's inner frustrations is to indicate summarily how one felt, but not to leave it at that. Add an attempt at self-analysis. For example, after noting "I felt hurt and that I was not understood", try to reflect about that in an objective way: "I think there were perhaps reasons for feeling hurt, but I was over-sensitive to that treatment; I behaved like a child", or "In my feelings, there was clearly an element of hurt, childish pride", and the like. The "diary" can also serve as a notebook for insights that sometimes come quite unexpectedly. *Resolutions* one has taken are also important material, especially as writing them down makes them all the more concrete and firm. Registered emotions, thoughts, and behaviors, however, are solely a means to an end, namely, better self-insight. Thinking them over eventually leads to better discernment of one's *motives* (especially those that are infantile or ego-centered).

Points of attention

Self-knowledge often comes about by taking a closer look at feelings and thoughts that are either unpleasant and/or agitating. When they occur, search yourself as to their meaning; what made you feel like that? Such negative feelings would include loneliness, rejection, abandonment, hurt, humiliation, worthlessness, listlessness, apathy, sadness or depression, agitation, nervousness, fear and anxiety, feelings of being chased, feelings of indignation, anger, jealousy, embitterment, longing, insecurity, doubt, and so on, and especially any feelings that strike you as somewhat extraordinary, as disturbing, peculiar, remarkable, or upsetting. Feelings having to do with the neurotic complex are usually associated with feeling *inadequate*, that is, one no longer feels master of oneself, one is out of balance. Why did I feel the way I did? Especially important questions to ask oneself are: "Was my inner reaction that of a 'child'?" and "Is a 'poor me' expressing itself here?" In fact, it turns out that many such feelings are childish frustrations, hurt pride, self-pity. The ensuing insight is: "I am inwardly not reacting as the mature man or

woman I can be, but more like a child, a teenager." In trying
to imagine what one's facial expression must have been, how
one's voice must have sounded, what the impression of one's
emotional expression must have been on others, one can perhaps see more clearly the concrete "inner child" one has formerly been. Some emotional reactions and behavioral habits
may easily be recognized as the actions of the "child" ego,
but it can be difficult to see childishness in other frustrated
feelings or impulses in spite of their being experienced as
troublesome, undesirable, or compulsive. *Displeasure* is the
most common indicator that something infantile is going on.
It often points to some manifestation of self-pity.

But how does one distinguish infantile from normal, ad-
equate, adult displeasure? In general, (1) noninfantile sorrow
and complaints do not primarily concern one's importance;
(2) nor do they as a rule bring a person completely out of
balance, a certain inner self-mastery remains; and (3) except
in extraordinary situations, they are not accompanied by an
overwhelming emotionality either. On the other hand, certain reactions may consist of both infantile and mature com-
ponents. A frustration, a loss, or hurt may be painful in itself,
even if one reacts to it as a child. If one cannot see if or how
far a reaction stems from the "child", it is better to drop the
incident for the moment. Later on, looking back at it after
some time, it may become clear.

One must scrutinize oneself with regard to certain social
behaviors. This concerns ways of relating to others: being
overly pleasing, servile, stubborn, hostile, suspicious, arrogant,
clinging, protecting or protection-seeking, leaning on other
people, being dominant, tyrannizing, hard, indifferent, critical, manipulative, aggressive, vengeful, fearful, avoiding or
provoking conflicts; being inclined to contradict negatively,
boasting and showing off, reacting with theatrical or dramatic behavior, being exhibitionistic and attention-seeking

(of which there are infinite variants) and so on. There are differentiations to be made here. One's behavior can differ depending on with whom one is dealing: others of the same or of the opposite sex; whether they are family members, friends, or colleagues; whether they are authorities or subordinates, strangers or people one knows well. Make notes of your observations and specify them according to the kind of social contacts to which they refer. Indicate which behaviors are most characteristic for you and your "child" ego.

One goal of this self-observation is to discover the *roles* one plays. These are roles of self-affirmation and getting attention in the majority of cases. One can act the successful one, the understanding one, the humorous one, the tragic figure, the sufferer, the helpless one, the faultless one, the important one (infinite variations). Role-playing, which betrays inner childishness, implies a measure of insincerity and inauthenticity; it may border on lying.

Verbal behavior, so typically human, can be very revealing too. The tone of voice itself may be informative, as with the young man who noticed how he drawled out his words, somewhat plaintively. "I believe I unconsciously take on a weak and babyish attitude, trying thereby to put others in the position of nice, understanding adults", was the result of his self-analysis. Another man observed that he was used to speaking in a dramatic tone to describe everything about his daily life and person, and indeed he tended to react a bit hysterically to the most common events.

Incidental observation of the *content* of one's verbal expressions can also be most instructive. Neurotic immaturity nearly always expresses itself in the tendency to complain— verbally and otherwise— about oneself, one's circumstances, others, life in general. And a considerable amount of ego-centeredness is manifest in the conversations and monologues of many persons with a homosexual neurosis as well.

"When I visit my friends, I can talk for more than an hour about myself," one homosexual client recognized, "while my attention wanders when my friend wants to tell me something, and then I can hardly listen to him." Such an observation is not exceptional at all. Ego-centeredness goes along with complaining. And many conversations of "neuroticistic" people end up in complaining. Record some of your informal conversations on tape and listen to them at least three times—a sometimes unflattering, instructive procedure!

What must be especially scrutinized are one's behaviors, attitudes, and thoughts with respect to one' *parents*. One may be—as far as the "child" ego is concerned—clinging, rebellious, contemptuous, fostering rivalry, rejecting, attention- (or admiration-) seeking, dependent, (overly) critical, and so on. This applies even if the parent(s) is (are) dead; one's infantile attitude of overattachment or hostility and accusation may remain alive in spite of that! Differentiate between the observations of your relationships with your mother and your father. Remember that the "childish ego" almost certainly shows up in the relationship with one's parents, whether in external behavior or in thoughts and feelings.

The same self-observations must be made concerning one's spouse, homosexual partners, or fantasy-partners. Many childish habits manifest themselves in the latter area: childish attention-seeking, role-playing, clinging, parasitical, manipulating, jealousy-inspired actions, and so on. Be radically sincere with yourself in your self-observation notes in this field, for precisely here is an (understandable) wish to deny, not to see certain motives, to justify.

As to *yourself*, consider what thoughts you cherish about yourself (negative as well as positive). Identify self-bashing, overcritical attitudes toward yourself, self-denunciatory ideas, feelings of inferiority, and so on, but also self-congratulation, self-flattering imaginings, hidden self-admiration in some sense or another, daydreams about yourself, and so on. Check inner manifestations of self-dramatization and self-victimization in your thoughts, fantasies, and emotions. Can you detect in yourself sentimentality? melancholic moods? Is there any conscious wallowing in self-pity? or possible self-destructive wishes or behaviors? (This is known as "psychic masochism", that is, purposely doing what you know will cause you harm or wallowing in misery that is self-inflicted or self-sought.)

As to *sexuality*, observe your spontaneous fantasies and try to identify the traits of physical appearance, behavior, or personality that arouse your interest in a real or imagined partner. Then relate them to your own inferiority feelings according to the rule that the fascinating traits in another are exactly those in which one feels inferior oneself. Try to discover any childish admiration or idolizing in your consideration of prospective "friends". Also try to discern the act of *comparing yourself with the other* in those feelings of interest in another of the same sex and in the *painful* feeling that is mixed up with the lustful longing. In fact, this painful feeling or longing is the childish feeling, "I am not like him (her)", and thus is a *complaint* or a pitiable "I wish he (she) would pay attention to me, poor inferior creature!" To analyze feelings of homoerotic "love" may not be easy, however, it is necessary to recognize the self-seeking motive in these feelings, the seeking of a loving friend for *me*, like a child who wants to be babied, egocentrically. Note also the psychological occasions that give rise to sexual fantasies or masturbation. These often happen to be feelings of frustration, so that sexual wishes function as self-comfort for one's "poor me".

Attention must be given, furthermore, to the way one fulfills the masculine or feminine "role". Check if there are manifestations of fear and avoidance of activities and interests typical of your sex, and if you feel inferior in them. Do you have habits and interests that are not in conformity with your sex? Most of these cross-gender or atypical gender behaviors and interests are infantile roles, and, when one inspects them closely, it is often possible to recognize underlying or connected fears and feelings of inferiority. Also these gender nonconformities can be recognized as ego-centered, immature. For example, a woman could see that her demanding and dictatorial ways "resembled" her manner of self-affirmation in puberty, when she resorted to them in order to find a place for herself among the others, out of a feeling of "not belonging". This role, now her second nature (as this is aptly called), then struck her as a childish "me too" attitude. A homosexual man with outspoken (pseudo)feminine mannerisms observed that he was constantly aware of his behavior. His effeminate ways, he noticed, were closely connected to strong and generalized feelings of inferiority and to a lack of normal self-assertion. Another man learned to recognize his effeminate presentation and demeanor as related to two different attitudes: self-complacency in the infantile enjoyment of playing the role of the lovely, girlish mother's boy and fear (a feeling of inferiority) of assuming a stronger, more manly kind of self-assertion. It usually takes some time of observing oneself before such self-insights dawn upon a person. Incidentally, cross-gender habits are often reflected in hairstyle, clothing, and a variety of mannerisms in speech, gestures, gait, way of laughing, and so on.

Work is another useful point of attention. Is your daily work done with inner aversion and complaining or with pleasure and energy? With responsibility? Is it a way of immature self-affirmation? Is there much unjustified, exaggerated complaining about the work situation?

After some period of this self-observation, make a very short summary description of the most important traits and motives of your infantile self, or "inner child". In many cases a slogan may be helpful: "the helpless boy who constantly tries to get pity and support" or "the wronged girl whom nobody understands", and so forth. Concrete incidents from the past or present often can sharply illustrate the traits of this "boy" or "girl". Such memories contain a vivid picture of your "child of the past". They contain the "child" in a nutshell. Therefore we can regard them as *key memories*. They can be of great help at moments one has to visualize one's "child" in order to recognize present infantile behaviors or when one has to combat them. They are mental "photographs" of the "child ego within" that one carries with oneself, like pictures of one's family members or friends in one's wallet.

Describe your key memory.

Moral Self-Knowledge

So far, the categories of self-observation discussed here have dealt with rather concrete events, inner and behavioral. There is a second level of self-reflection, however, the psychological-moral level. To observe oneself from this viewpoint overlaps in part the type of psychological self-observations described above. But moral self-insight goes more to the roots of personality. Pragmatically speaking, psychological self-knowledge, which implies moral self-understanding, can greatly spur the motivation to change. We must remember Henri Baruk's splendid insight: "Moral consciousness is the cornerstone of our psyche" (1979, 291). How could that not have consequences for psychotherapy, and self-therapy or self-education?

Moral(-psychological) self-insights generally concern abstractions, i.e., rather constant inner attitudes, although these may be discovered through concrete behaviors. One man saw how he had childishly lied in a certain situation, out of fear of criticism. He recognized in this incident an attitude or habit of his ego that was even more basic than his habit of lying as a defense (out of fear of hurt for his ego), namely, his deeply rooted selfishness, his moral impurity ("sinfulness", the Christian would call it). This is a level of self-knowledge more fundamental than the purely psychological. It sets also free—precisely for that reason—more curative forces than can be done by mere psychological insights. But often we cannot draw the line between the psychological and the moral too sharply, because most sensible psychological self-insights touch the moral dimension (consider, for example, the recognition of childish self-pity). The interesting correlation is that many things we regard as "childish" are at the same time felt as morally worthy of reproof, sometimes even as immoral.

Selfishness is the common denominator of most, if not all, immoral habits and attitudes, "vices". Those habits are at one end of a bipolar spectrum; virtues, morally upright habits, form the opposite pole. For one who wants to investigate his neurotic complex, it is useful to observe himself for a while under the moral dimension as well. Suggested points of attention are the following:

1. contentment versus discontentment (related, of course, to the tendency to indulge in complaining);
2. courage versus cowardice (note the concrete situations or areas of behavior where you notice particularities);
3. perseverance, firmness versus weakness, being weak-willed, avoidance of hardship, softness to self;
4. temperance versus lack of self-discipline, self-indulgence, self-pampering (lack of self-restriction can be one's vice in eating, drinking, talking, working, or lust—of which there are many kinds);
5. diligence, industriousness versus laziness (in any area);

6. humility, realism toward oneself versus pride, arrogance, vanity, pedantry (specify area of behavior);
7. modesty versus immodesty;
8. honesty and sincerity versus dishonesty, insincerity, and habits of lying (specify);
9. reliability versus unreliability (with respect to persons, matters, promises);
10. responsibility (normal sense of duties) versus irresponsibility (with respect to family, friends, persons, work, tasks);
11. understanding, forgiveness versus vengefulness, vindictiveness, embitterment, destructiveness (as to family members, friends, colleagues, others);
12. normal enjoyment of possessions versus greed (specify manifestations).

A basic question for anyone searching his motivational life is: Judging by my preoccupations and interests, what is *in fact* my main or ultimate goal(s) in life? Are they directed toward self or toward others, to tasks, ideals, objective values? (Goals directed toward self include money and possessions, power, fame, social recognition, attention and/or esteem from others, a comfortable life, eating, drinking, sex.)

8

QUALITIES TO CULTIVATE

Beginning the Battle:
Hope, Self-Discipline, Sincerity

Growing self-insight is the first step in any change. During the therapy process (which is a battle), self-insight continues to grow, along with improvement. One may yet see a good many more things, but after some time insights will deepen.

Initial self-insight into the dynamics of one's neurosis gives one one's bearings, and this arouses *hope*. Hope is a positive and healthy, antineurotic mind-set. It can, in some cases, make problems much easier, even make them disappear for a while. The foundation of the habits that constitute the neurosis, however, is still there, so, in all likelihood, symptoms will reappear. Hope must be cherished throughout the process of change nevertheless. Hope is based on realism: however often neurotic—or, for that matter, homosexual— feelings may present themselves, however often one may give in to them, as long as there is a constant effort to improve, one will see positive achievements. Moods of despair are part of the game, at least in many cases, but one must curtail them, keep calm, and go on. Realistic hope is quiet optimism, not agitated euphoria.

The next step is indispensable: *self-discipline*. For the most part, this concerns trivial things: waking up on time; keeping regular habits in taking care of one's body, in one's meals, clothing, hair; putting a reasonable order into the small affairs of everyday life and work, not delaying works or business that deserve priority; planning (roughly, not meticulously or obsessively) the day, one's amusement, social life. If there are points of shaky or absent self-discipline, note them and begin working on them. Many homosexually inclined people have difficulty with some form of self-discipline. To disregard these problems, hoping for an emotional cure that will solve everything else, is foolish. No (self-)therapy can satisfactorily succeed if this down-to-earth dimension of daily self-discipline is neglected. Invent simple methods for your characteristic weak spots. Start with one or two areas of failing self-discipline; when they improve, the rest will follow more easily.

It is only logical that *sincerity* is obligatory. Sincerity to oneself, in the first place. This means training oneself to pay unprejudiced attention to what is going on in one's mind, to one's motives and real intentions, including the promptings of one's conscience. Sincerity means not arguing away the perceptions or intuitions of one's so-called "better self", but trying to put them in straightforward, simple words so as to become maximally aware of them. (Make a habit of writing down important thoughts and self-perceptions.)

Sincerity, moreover, means taking courage to communicate one's weaknesses and failures to another person who, either as therapist or guide/coach, is there to help. Virtually everyone has the tendency to conceal certain aspects of his intentions and feelings, both from himself and from others, yet it is not only liberating to overcome this hurdle but also indispensable for progress.

To the requirements of sincerity, the Christian would add sincerity toward God, in one's searching of conscience as well as in prayer and conversation with him. Insincerity toward him would be, for example, asking for his help without at least trying to do what one can do oneself—irrespective of the outcome.

In view of the self-tragedizing tendency of the neurotic mind, it is important to warn that sincerity is not theatrical, but sober, simple, and straightforward.

Fighting Neurotic Self-Pity; Humor

After recognizing, in everyday life, a momentary or more chronic manifestation of the "inner complaining child", the procedure to follow is to imagine this "poor me child/teen-ager" standing before you in the flesh. Or imagine that your adult ego has been replaced by the "child ego" so only your adult body is present. Then mentally represent this "child" as acting or reacting, or just thinking and feeling, in the concrete situation in which you find yourself. To represent the "child" well, you might use the "key memory", the mental "photograph" of your "child ego" (see p. 110).

This recognition of one's inner and/or outward behavior as embodied in a "child" can be rather easy. It appears easy when someone can say, for instance: "I felt completely like a little boy (who was rejected, criticized, not esteemed; who felt pitifully lonely, humiliated, fearful in front of an authority figure, or angry, rebellious, and so on)." It can also be easy for someone else who observed the person's behavior to tell him: "You behaved like a child." But often acknowledgment is not easy, for two reasons. First, there can be considerable resistance to seeing oneself as *merely* a "child". "My feelings are more serious and worthwhile than that"; "Perhaps I was somewhat childish, nevertheless, I actually had good reasons for feeling agitated and hurt. . . ." In short, *childish pride* can prevent one from seeing oneself in so simple a light. Second, emotions and inner reactions can often be rather confusing.

One does not clearly discern what one is really thinking, feeling, or willing; and it may also be unclear what element of the situation or others' behavior provoked the inner reaction. As for the first difficulty, sincerity will help, and for the second, reflection, analysis, reasoning. Make a note of unintelligible reactions and discuss them with your therapist or coach; his observations or critical questions may be an aid. If this doesn't solve the problem satisfactorily either, it is best to drop the incident for the time being. In the course of self-analysis and self-treatment, when one has become better aware of one's "inner child's" typical patterns of reaction, incidents of "insoluble" "child" reactions will occur less frequently.

There will be instances enough, however, when the complaints of the "child", and the childish quality of one's inner and/or outward reactions, are visible. Sometimes merely recognizing the "poor child" is sufficient to create an inner distance to childish feelings and self-pity. The unpleasant feeling need not disappear completely to lose its urgency.

At other times, it is appropriate to see the irony of the "poor me", for instance, by saying to the "inner child", the childish self, such comments as "Oh, how sad, how pitiful!" or "Poor you!" If it works, this method produces a weak smile, especially if one can imagine one's face as that of the child-of-the-past, with a pathetic expression. This method can be modified according to one's individual taste and sense of humor. Make little jokes at your infantile self. Still better, if the opportunity presents itself, make such jokes in front of others—when two people laugh, the effect is doubled.

With stronger and more obsessive complaints (especially those associated with rejection, such as hurt childish pride, feelings of worthlessness, ugliness, and inferiority; physical complaints, such as tiredness; or distress over injustice suffered or adverse circumstances), apply the method of *hyperdramatization* devised by psychiatrist Arndt. It consists of exaggerating the tragic or dramatic aspects of the infantile complaint until it becomes ridiculous, until one reacts by smiling or even laughing. This method was used intuitively by the famous seventeenth-century French playwright Molière when he suffered from bouts of obsessive hypochondria. In response to his own obsession, he produced a comedy with a hero who so exaggeratedly dramatized his sufferings and "imagined illnesses" that it made the public (and himself as well) laugh heartily.

Laughing is a very good remedy against neurotic emotions. But it takes courage and some practice before one can say ridiculous things about and to "oneself" (that is, one's childish ego), make ridiculous representations of "oneself", or purposely make faces at "oneself" in the mirror, imitating oneself, one's behavior, one's plaintive voice comically, making fun of oneself, of one's hurt feelings. The neurotic ego takes itself very seriously—at any rate, it takes its complaints tragically; the person may otherwise have a well-developed sense of humor in nonsensitive areas of his personality.

Hyperdramatization is a basic technique of self-humor. But any other form of self-humor is welcome. What is the purpose? In general, humor serves to reveal the relativity of one's feeling important or tragic; to counteract complaining and self-pity, so that one can better accept what is inevitable and "suffer without complaining" when things, big or small, just are the way they are; and to help one become more realistic, to see the true proportions of oneself and others, that is, to come out of one's excessively subjective or imagined perception of the world and of others.

In hyperdramatizing complaints, one talks to one's "child", imagined as within or standing before one. For instance, when self-pity arises over unfriendly treatment or some kind of rejection, one might address the inner child in this way: "Poor 'Johnny', how harshly you've been treated! Beaten up, all bloody, with your clothes all torn. . . ." When feeling hurt childish pride, one might say, "You poor thing, your statue in a majestic pose, quite like a little Napoleon, has been hauled down like Lenin's after the fall of communism", while imagining the jeering mob and one's poor "child" coming down, in ropes, crying. To self-pity over loneliness—a highly frequent complaint among homosexuals—one might respond, "Such agony! Your shirt is wet, even the windows are steamed by your tears, and the sheets of your bed are dripping, saturated with your tears; a pond of tears is forming on the floor; fishes with an intensely sad look are swimming aimless circles in it"; and so on.

Many homosexuals, both male and female, feel uglier than others of the same sex, though they find it painful to admit. Feelings of ugliness can be met with an exaggeration of the bodily aspect (being skinny, fat, having big ears, big nose, narrow shoulders, and so on) that is central to the complaint. To counteract comparing yourself negatively to other, "more attractive", males or females, represent your "child" as a poor beggar boy or girl, abandoned by everyone, crippled, with pathetically old and worn clothes. A man might imagine himself an ugly, crying, babyish creature without muscles or any physical strength at all, with an extremely high, shrill, little voice, and so on. A woman might imagine an ugly, supermasculine "girl", with a beard, biceps like Popeye's, and so on. The next step would be to contrast this poor one with the fascinating "idol", exaggerating the radiance of the other, and then to imagine the piercing cry for love on the part of the "poor me", who dies in the street after the other has passed by without even having perceived the love-hungry little pariah.

As a variant, invent a fantasy scene in which the yearning "boy" or "girl" is taken in the arms of the adored lover, while the moon cries from sheer emotion, "Finally, a bit of love after all these sufferings!" And imagine this scene—filmed by a hidden camera—being represented in the cinema: the public cries and sobs without interruption, they come out broken, crying in each other's arms over this poor "boy" or "girl" who, after so much and such terrible searching for a bit of warmth, has found it in the end. This way, the tragic love-craving of the "child" ego is superdramatized. In hyper-dramatization one can proceed as one likes; sometimes the fantasy takes on a life of its own, concocting whole stories. Use whatever may seem humorous to you; invent your own brand of "self"-irony.

If one objects, as is often done, that these are silly or childish things, I agree. They are tricks. Usually, however, such objections stem from an inner resistance to laughing at oneself. My advice, then, is to start with small, innocent jokes about frustrations that are not felt as particularly serious. Humor can work well, and, although this is childish humor, we must not lose sight of the fact that it is also childish emotionality that is being fought with this trick. The use of self-irony and self-humor presupposes, however, at least in part, insight into the infantile or pubertal character of these reactions. The first step is always recognition of and admission of infantilism and self-pity. Incidentally, it is an interesting fact that self-humor is habitual in humble and psychologically healthy people.

The field of verbal behavior is excellent in the detection and combat of complaining tendencies. One can complain mentally or in words, in speech. A good exercise is to note one's words during a conversation with friends or colleagues and mentally register every time the urge to complain crops up. Try not to satisfy this urge: change the subject or say something like "It is difficult (or mean, unjust, and so on), *but* okay; we must see how we can make the best of it." Conducting this simple experiment now and then can reveal how strong the tendency to complain about one's fate and frustrations really is and how frequently and easily one gives in to it. It is also a good practice to withstand an urge to "co-complain" when others are complaining, expressing their indignation or discontentment.

Anticomplaining therapy, by the way, is not a simplistic variant of "positive thinking". There is nothing wrong with expressing sorrow and everyday frustrations to friends or family members if it is done soberly, with the necessary perspective on the relativity of one's complaints. Normal negative emotions and thoughts need not be denied by exaggerated "positive thinking"; our adversary is infantile, childish self-pity alone. One can *hear* the difference between normal expressions of grief and disappointment and childish whining, harping, lamenting.

"But it takes strength and courage to suffer and not to indulge in infantile self-pity and complaining!" one might aptly remark. Indeed, we are talking about a struggle that is more than a mobilization of one's capacity for humor. The most important thing is to work at it steadily, one day at a time.

Patience and Humility

Working steadily brings us to the virtue of *patience*. Patience with one's failures and with the gradual element of progress. Impatience is an attribute of youth. A child does not easily accept his weaknesses, and when he wants to change something, he feels it must happen overnight. Conversely, healthy self-acceptance (which is quite different from the currently propagated indulgence of one's weaknesses) means doing one's very best, while calmly accepting oneself as the weak and often failing little person one is. In other words, self-acceptance stands for realism with respect to the self, for *humility*.

Humility is central to the mature personality. It is an objective reality that each human person *has* his frailties and often considerable imperfections, psychological as well as moral. To imagine oneself a hero is childish thinking; consequently, it is childish to live a tragic role—otherwise formulated, to do so would constitute a lack of humility. Karl Stern asserted: "The so-called 'inferiority complex' and true humility are two opposites" (1951, 97). Exercising the virtuous habit of humility strongly combats neurosis. And practicing self-humor, a means of seeing the relativity of the infantile ego and challenging its claim of being important, can be regarded as an exercise in humility.

Inferiority complexes are usually accompanied by heightened superiority feelings in some area or other. The childish ego tries to prove its worth; not being able to accept its alleged inferiority, it is carried away by self-pity. Children are by nature ego-centered and thus feel important, the center of the world. Therefore, they are inclined to (infantile, because they are children) pride. In a sense, in any inferiority complex lies an element of hurt pride insofar as the inner child cannot accept his (perceived) inferiority. This makes the ensuing efforts at overcompensation understandable. ("Actually, I am special, better than the rest.") This in turn explains the lack of humility in neurotic self-affirmation, role-playing, and in the tendency to be the center of attention and sympathy. Deeply hurt self-esteem is even akin to delusions of grandeur.

Many homosexuals, male as well as female, demonstrate overcompensatory arrogance. From their feelings of inferiority, their childhood complex of "not belonging", they developed airs of superiority: "I am not one of you; *actually* I am better than you, special. I have a superior nature: I am specially gifted, specially sensitive. Specially tragic." The way to adopting superior roles has sometimes been paved by special attention and valuing from a parent, usually, in homosexuals, the opposite-sex parent. The boy who was mother's favorite or admired son is likely to develop ideas of superiority, as will the girl whose head has been turned by her father's special attention and praise. Arrogance in many homosexuals can be traced to their tender years.

In combination with feelings of inferiority, arrogance makes such homosexuals vulnerable to criticisms and easily insulted. Men and women with a homosexual complex who have decided that their desires are "natural" often succumb to an impulse to equate their being different with being superior. For, in the last analysis, they do not consider themselves equal to "common" heterosexuals, but superior to them. The same can be said for pedophiliacs; André Gide glorified his "love" for boys as the most superb variant of human tenderness. Not only is it theoretically true that these homosexuals are inspired by pride in reversing what is unnatural and natural, in calling right what is wrong, but their pride is also visible in their whole behavior. "I was the King", an ex-homosexual once said of his former lifestyle. They are vainglorious, narcissistic in demeanor and clothing; some even border on megalomania. Some despise ordinary mankind, ordinary marriage, ordinary families. Their arrogance blinds them to many values, and certainly to the insight that they are but pitiable children, devoid of wisdom.

Learning humility is liberating. It is done by discovering thoughts, expressions, and impulses of vanity, arrogance, superiority, self-congratulation, and boasting, as well as hurt pride and unacceptance of well-intentioned criticisms—and by refuting such thoughts, mildly satirizing them, or otherwise rejecting them. It is done by building a new self-image, that of the real self, who indeed has capabilities, but capabilities that are limited, and who himself is on the whole but an average, modest human being, nothing very special.

9

CHANGING PATTERNS
OF THOUGHT AND BEHAVIOR

Fighting Homosexual Feelings

The interior battle against homosexual inclinations mobilizes the faculties of self-insight and the will. The aspect of will is indispensable. It means that as long as homosexual longing or fantasy is cherished—despite good intentions to the contrary—it is hardly possible to weaken the homosexual interest. For, regardless of the wish to get rid of it, that interest is nourished every time one secretly or consciously gives in to enjoying it. The comparison with the urges of alcoholism or, to a degree, of a smoking addiction is to the point. Emphasizing the will does not mean that certain self-insights are not very helpful. But, by themselves, insights usually lack the power to overcome the infantile lustful erotic impulse; it is only by a total effort of the will that this impulse can be silenced in a concrete situation. This effort should be made in all quietude, without panic, with the attitude of the adult who tries to control a difficult situation: patiently, realistically. Don't let yourself be intimidated by the impulse, don't make a drama of it, don't deny it, and don't exaggerate the annoyance it causes you either. Then try to say "No" to it.

The faculty of the will is generally underestimated, for in

modern psychotherapy we are used to giving a one-sided emphasis to both intellectual insights (psychoanalysis) and training (behavior therapy, psychology of learning). And yet it is precisely the will that is central; insights and training are necessary, but their effectiveness depends on a correct orientation of the will.

By inner reflection, the homosexual must reach a full decision of the will: I shall leave absolutely no room whatsoever for these homosexual impulses. He must gradually grow in that decision. He must consider it often, especially at moments of calm, when clear thinking is not clouded by erotic excitement. Once the decision is made, he will reject even slight occasions for homosexual excitation or homoerotic enjoyment, immediately and totally—not half-heartedly. In the vast majority of cases in which a homosexual is "willing" but has little success, this is due to a will that is not completely decided; for that reason, he is unable to fight vigorously and will be inclined to blame the strength of his homosexual orientation or "the circumstances" for his poor results rather than the incompleteness of his decision. After several years of relative success and periodical relapses into homosexual fantasy, a homosexual man discovered that he had never really and fully willed to get free of his lust. "Now it was clear to me why it had been so difficult. I had wanted it, certainly, but never one hundred percent." The first struggle is therefore to strive for a purified will. That achieved, one must renew the decision quite regularly, so that it becomes stable, a habit. If not, the decision will surely weaken again.

It is essential to recognize that there will be moments or hours when the sound will is under heavy attack by lustful longing. "At such moments I ultimately want to consent to my longings with my will", many clients with otherwise good intentions have to admit. Then the struggle is really painful; it is all the more so, however, if one does not possess a firm will beforehand.

The impulse may be to fantasize about a person met in the street or at the office, seen on television or in the newspaper; it may be a daydream aroused by certain thoughts or experiences in everyday life. Or it may be an impulse to go out to seek a partner in some meeting place. Deciding "No", therefore, has varied grades of difficulty. The desires may be so strong that they confuse clear thinking, and then one has to act on the power of the will alone. Of help at these moments of tension are two thoughts: "I must be sincere" and "I am free, even under the pressure of this burning desire." Sincerity here means recalling, "I *know* I must resist, so I must not deceive myself." To exercise freedom of will is to recognize, "I can lift my hand; I can walk away, if I give a command, at this very moment. So it is also in my power to stay here, in this room, and show myself master of my impulses. If I want to drink, I can decide not to and accept the thirst." Small tricks can be helpful, such as saying aloud, "I am deciding to stay at home", or writing down some helpful thoughts and reading these at a moment of emergency.

It is easier quietly to avert a gaze, to cut off a train of imaginings, not to dwell on the sight of a person or picture. The will is facilitated by insight. Try to see that, in looking at that person, you may be making a *comparison*: "He is a Prince Charming, she is a goddess, and I am pitifully inferior by comparison." Try to recognize that the impulse is one of pathetic craving by the infantile ego: "You are so beautiful, so manly (so feminine). Please, pay attention to poor me!" The more one is aware of this "poor me" attitude, the easier it is to distance oneself from it and to use the weapon of one's will.

An important aid is seeing how childish this seeking homoerotic contacts—in reality or fantasy—really is. Try to perceive that in such a longing you are not a mature, responsible person, but a child who wants to pamper himself, getting warmth and sensual pleasure for himself. Understand that this is not real love, but self-seeking, in which the partner is more an object of pleasure than a person. This should also be considered at times when the sexual wish is absent.

Clearer awareness of the childish, egotistical nature of homosexual satisfaction, moreover, opens the eyes to its moral impurity. Lust blurs the moral perception of purity and impurity, but not altogether; many do think that their homosexual behavior with other persons or their masturbatory practices are impure. To enhance this awareness, one must reinforce the will to resist; one's healthy emotions detest one's impurity. Never mind that this view may be ridiculed by those committed to their homosexuality. They are simply not honest. Everyone can decide to see or not to see the qualities of purity and impurity. Refusing to see them is a defense mechanism: "denial". A highly infantile client, whose homosexual desires centered on sniffing at young men's underwear while imagining sexual games with them, was helped by the thought that occurred to him, that his behavior was sneaky. He felt, in fact, that he misused the bodies of his friends in his fantasy while misusing their underwear only for his own sensual gratification. The idea made him feel impure, foul. It is in this field as with many other immoral actions: the greater the inner moral disapproval (in other words, the clearer the perception of the action's moral ugliness), the better one can say "No".

Homosexual arousal is often a reaction of self-comfort after disappointment or feelings of displeasure. In such cases, the inherent self-pity must be recognized and hyperdramatized. Adversity taken well usually does not elicit erotic fantasies. However, homosexual impulses occasionally appear at quite different moments, when one is feeling fine and well and not thinking along such lines at all. In that case, they are provoked by memories, associations. One finds oneself in a situation formerly connected with homosexual adventures—in a certain city, at a certain place, on a special day, and the like. All of a sudden the impulse is there, one is taken unprepared. But then, if one knows such moments from experience, it is certainly possible to prepare oneself, among other things, by regularly repeating the decision not to surrender to the sudden fascination of these special circumstances or environments.

Many homosexual men and women are addicted to the practice of masturbation, which chains them to their immature interests and sexual ego-centeredness. The battle with this habit can be won provided one perseveres, relapses notwithstanding. There is, of course, a big overlap with the attempts to overcome homoerotic imagery, but there are some specific points to be made here.

For many, masturbation is a form of self-comfort after disappointment or frustration. One lets oneself sink into infantile imagery. A good strategy is to make a firm proposal, every morning, and repeat it whenever necessary (in the evening or before going to bed): "The next part of the day (night) I shall not give in." With such a mind-set, the first signs of the emerging desire are better recognized. Then one may say to oneself: "I will not give myself this pleasure; rather, I will accept the little suffering it means not to get what I want." Imagine a child whose mother refuses to give it candy—the child may grow furious, or start crying and perhaps even kicking. Then *hyperdramatize* your childish ego as if it were behaving that way ("I want my candy!"). Or say, "How pitiful that you won't get your little comfort." Or treat yourself (that is, your child-ego) as a stern father would: "No, little Johnny (Mary), Daddy says 'No' today. No more little games. Perhaps tomorrow. And you do what your daddy says." And tomorrow, do the same. So, concentrate on today, don't think: "I will never be able to overcome this, never be able to stop doing this." The struggle must be daily; in this way, abstinence builds up. Also, don't dramatize weak moments and relapses. Say to yourself, "It was stupid, but we go on", like a sportsman. Then one will see that one grows stronger, relapses or not. And it is a liberation, like weaning from alcohol; one feels better, more peaceful, happier.

Another trick: imagine yourself as *not giving in* at the moment of the impulse, as a mature person who feels the impulse, yet firmly goes on with his work or quietly lies in bed and remains master of himself. Imagine yourself as vividly as possible as such a mature person who spurs the will not to indulge. "Yes, that's the person I would like to be!" Or imagine having to tell your wife or husband—your possible spouse in the future—or your (future) children whether or not you fought this masturbation impulse like a responsible person. Imagine having to tell them you did not fight, or hardly fought, like a weakling, and how ashamed you would be in front of them.

Concerning *hyperdramatization*, one may hyperdramatize the "fulfillment" of "love" in masturbation fantasies. For instance, tell your "inner child" (or, for that matter, yourself when you see that at this moment your ego has become again an adolescent): "He looked deep into your eyes, expressing eternal love for you, poor boy (girl), and warmth for your abandoned and love-hungry soul", and so on. In general, try to ridicule and satirize your fantasies or their elements (for instance, fetishist peculiarities). But first and foremost hyperdramatize the—perhaps hardly conscious—craving, yearning, self-dramatizing complaint: "Give me, poor, little ol' me, your *love*!" Homoerotic fantasies, like the masturbation impulses connected with them, give way to humor, to the act of smiling.

The problem with neurotic emotions is that they make the person allergic to self-humor. The infantile ego resists "attacks" of humor and jokes directed against its self-importance. Nevertheless, self-humor can be learned by training.

It is logical that some homosexuals have infantile ideas about sexuality. So some may think that masturbation is necessary to train their sexual virility. Of course, the masculinity inferiority complex implicit in it must be hyperdramatized. Never "prove" your masculinity by muscle training, body-building, nurturing beards and mustaches, whatever. To do so would be counterproductive in that it would feed a pubertal mentality.

The believing Christian must also resort to prayer. Prayer can be most effective in overcoming these sexual fantasies and masturbation impulses. But this does not exclude the struggle of the will we dealt with above. First, because it must not only be prayer in general, but prayer at the crucial moments when the impulses present themselves. The interesting observation one can make here is that many religious persons with a homosexual complex, although they do pray at other times, refuse to do so at the very moment of "temptation". To pray under these circumstances requires an effort of the will. If this is made, and the person tries earnestly to apply the available methods, yet still feels incapable of overcoming a strong impetus to go after a partner, to masturbate, to indulge in homoerotic daydreaming, he will notice that an honest prayer with the mind-set of a son addressing a good Father will keep him from succumbing. One who really tries to do what he can and then sincerely asks for help will experience it, subtly, but unmistakably.

A believing Catholic will also have recourse to the Blessed Virgin, whose intercession with God is particularly effective in matters of chastity, to the saints, and to his guardian angel. He will be inwardly strengthened by the sacraments of confession and of the Eucharist. American Catholics with homosexual problems can find encouragement and support from a sound religious approach that does not shun the notion of "chastity" at one of the chapters of the organization Courage, founded by Fr. John Harvey (see Harvey 1987, 1996). Active membership in this organization and (self-) therapy as described in this book are not antagonistic, but complementary. Moreover, regular small physical mortifications prove helpful in the battle with sexual obsessions, especially when they are offered up to God, as I have heard from Catholic and Protestant clients alike. Remarkable that this old wisdom seems practically forgotten.

The ideal for the future treatment of homosexuality for Christians will be an interplay between psychological and spiritual elements and procedures. Such an approach, Christian and psychological, is, on the whole, the best guarantee for change.

With respect to prayer, I recommend this advice from a powerful modern spiritual author, J. Escrivá, which can be of support and comfort to the one whose resolution and hope for a change waver now and then: "The first thing needed as far as prayer is concerned is to keep at it; the second thing is to be humble. Have a holy stubbornness, be trusting. Remember that when we ask the Lord for something important, He may want to be asked for many years. Keep on! But keep on with ever increasing trust" (1988, 194).

Fighting the Infantile Ego

So this is the immature, ego-centered "self". The reader who has thought over the various statements in the chapter on self-knowledge (chapter 7) will perhaps have noted several of his own infantile traits or needs that came to mind. Now,

growing to emotional maturity does not proceed automatically; one must wage the battle with the infantile ego (and
take the time for it).

The homosexually inclined person will do well to focus
on his "inner child's" *seeking attention and sympathy*. Its variants are trying to be important, respected, esteemed, loved,
pitied, or admired. Its numerous ramifications must be detected in everyday life and in one's contacts with others, and
its enjoyments of this kind must be denied. More and more,
it will become clear how many acts, thoughts, and motives
spring from the infantile need for self-affirmation (which is
different from a healthy joy in functioning and self-realiza-
tion). The infantile ego strives after exclusive attention from
other people. Its need for love and sympathy may be tyranni-
cal; it is easily hurt, jealous when others get the attention.
The "inner child's" drive for love and attention must be dis-
tinguished from the normal human need for love. The latter
is, at least partially, subordinated to the need to love other
persons. For example, mature love that is rejected responds
with sadness, not so much with indignation and infantile self-
pity.

Any kind of infantile self-affirmation should be "frustrated"; in this way, swift progress can be made. Don't forget
attempts to be "great" in one's own eyes, to excel, to be
admirable. In a sense, infantile self-affirmation seems "reparative", particularly to inferiority complaints. In effect,
however, it merely nourishes such complaints as it strengthens one's ego-centeredness (all infantile urges and emotions
interconnect like communicating vessels; feeding one automatically strengthens the others). Mature self-affirmation,
which provides a different kind of joy, is contentment with
being able to achieve something, not, however, because "*I*
am so special"; partly, it is gratefulness. The mature adult is
aware of the relativity of his achievements.

Role-playing; pretending; trying to make an interesting or special impression—these behaviors are part of the category of "attention/sympathy-seeking". Frustrating these tendencies by stopping them as soon as one notices them costs a little, for one gives up the emotional rewards of a tickled narcissism. The result, however, is a feeling of relief, liberation; one feels inwardly more independent, stronger. The role-player, the attention-seeker, conversely, makes himself dependent on others' judgments of him.

Besides being vigilant against these behaviors and stopping them when they present themselves, one must work at the positive side as well, namely, by *serving*. With this concept what is meant first is considering, in all kinds of situations and occupations, one's *tasks* and *duties*. It means asking oneself the simple question: What should or could be my contribution in this situation (whether it be a meeting, a celebration in the family, daily work, or an entertainment situation)? The "inner child", conversely, is preoccupied with the questions: "What's in it for *me*? How can I profit from this situation; what can the others do for *me*? What impression can I make on them?" and so on, thus I-related thinking. To counteract this, a purposeful effort to accomplish what one thinks might be one's contribution to or meaning for *others* proves most helpful. The ego-centered person who, apart from normally enjoying a meeting with friends or colleagues, consciously tries to be of some value to the others, in fact, redirects his ego-centeredness, will feel more contented on the way. To phrase it differently, the question is What are—as I can see them—my smaller and greater *responsibilities*? One must specify these in relation to one's long-term goals as well as to everyday situations of short duration. Moreover, what are my responsibilities in friendships, in my work, my marriage, to my children, to my health, my body, my leisure time? These questions may seem trivial. Yet the homosexually preoccupied husband who only lamented about his anguishing dilemma, choosing between "family or friend", and eventually left his family for his lover, in reality had not honestly reflected on his responsibilities. He rather repressed the thought of them, smothering it in self-pity about his tragic predicament.

To be no longer a child psychologically is the goal of any neurosis therapy. Negatively put, this implies that one tries not to live exclusively for oneself, for the glory of the infantile ego, or for its pleasures. Insofar as one succeeds with that, homosexual interests will diminish. The crucial thing, however, is first to see one's behavior and motives under the light of childishness and being directed to self. "I seem to care only for myself", an otherwise sincere homosexual man concluded; "I do not know what loving is." Infantile selfishness appears to be the essence of the homosexual liaison as well: wanting a friend for *oneself*. "That is why I am always domineering and demanding in a relation with a girl", a lesbian woman acknowledged. "She must be fully *mine*." Many homosexuals *feign* warmth and love for their partners and delude themselves into believing these sentiments are real, but in effect they cherish a self-serving sentimentality and play a game. Time and again it turns out that they can be hard on their partners and basically disinterested in them. This love is self-deception.

A man who was very generous to his many friends, buying them extravagant presents, helping them with money when they were in need, actually did not give away anything. He bought their sympathy. Another realized that he was constantly preoccupied with his physical appearance, spending practically all the money he earned on clothes, hairstylists, colognes. (Of course) he felt physically inferior and unattractive, and as a result inwardly pitied himself, but his over-compensatory *narcissism* was *pseudo-reparative* selfishness. A teenager may be expected to be preoccupied with styling his hair for some time, but then, when he grows up, he will accept it the way it is, and the subject is no longer of much relevance to him. Not so for many homosexual men: they cling to their childish, wishful thinking about their imagined beauty, contemplate themselves a long time in the mirror or watch themselves in their imagination as they walk in the street or deal with other people. Self-humor is a good antidote for such behavior (e.g., "Boy, do you look wonderful!").

There are all kinds of narcissism. A lesbian woman who behaves too much like a man may childishly enjoy her role, as does the homosexual man who half-consciously cultivates pseudofeminine ways, or, in another case, childishly plays a supermasculine role. "How terrific I am" is the unspoken, accompanying thought.

Exercising love for the other people in one's environment may be felt as frustrating. Only one's "me" is interesting, not others. Learning to love begins with cultivating an interest in the other person: How does he live, what does he feel, what will objectively be good for him? From this inner attention small gestures and deeds result; one begins feeling more responsible for others. (But not in the way some neurotic people do, feeling obliged to take the whole life of others on their shoulders. This kind of taking responsibility for others may be another form of egocentricity: *I* am the important one upon whom rests the world's fate.) With a healthy concern for others, feelings of love come into being, as a consequence of restructured thinking and attention.

Many homosexuals are arrogant, occasionally or chronically, in their demeanor; others chiefly in their thoughts (e.g., "I am better than you"). Such thoughts must be caught the moment they cross the mind and then cut off, or satirized, made humorous. As the "inner child's" self-importance diminishes, some narcissistic satisfactions disappear, such as subconscious ideas of being special, a genius, superior. Nietzschean superman illusions are childish thinking; what is the reverse? A healthy recognition of one's not being better than others; an ability to laugh at oneself.

Jealousy is childish as well. "He has this or that, *I don't*! And I can't stand it! Poor me!" He is more beautiful, stronger, more boyish, more athletic, more popular, he has more flair; she is prettier, more charming, more girlish, more radiant, of a more graceful build, gets more attention from the boys. In looking thus at others of the same sex, the infantile ego's admiration and longing for contact is mixed up with jealousy. Neutralizing the voice of the "child" is the right action to take: "Okay, let him be much more perfect; I will try to be fully *content* with everything I am, physically and psychologically, even if I were the least, the most inferior, of my sex." Hyperdramatization of or satirizing the infantile ego's alleged inferior manly or feminine qualities may thereafter reinforce the attempt to view members of one's own sex in a less ego-centered way.

If the reader thinks over this issue of mature loving, he will come to the conclusion that, since overcoming homosexuality is equal to becoming more mature, this inner battle is a specific variant of the battle of every human to outgrow his personal areas of infantilism.

Mending the Sex Role

Becoming a mature man or woman also implies feeling at home in one's natural, inborn sex role. Not infrequently does a homosexual person cherish the wish, "If only I weren't obliged to be a grown-up!" The injunction "Behave like a man (like a lady)" sounds like a curse to them. They have difficulty imagining themselves as grown-ups because of their infantile complaint about gender inferiority. Besides, they often have an exaggerated, unrealistic view of manhood and womanhood. They feel more relaxed in the child role: "the nice, sweet, charming boy", "the helpless boy", "the girlish boy", or "the tomboyish girl", "the aggressive, manly girl", "the fragile, abandoned little girl". . . . They don't like to admit that these are false "selves", false identities. In them they seek comfort, a niche in social life. At the same time this role-playing may provide some (again, not all) with the narcissistic pleasure of feeling dramatic and "special".

The homosexual man may seek masculinity in his idolized partners, while at the same time he himself (or, rather, his "child" ego) can paradoxically be disdainful of masculinity, because he feels "more sensitive", superior to this "vulgar" manliness. This makes for the near-proverbial arrogance of some. The lesbian may despise femininity as an inferior quality—a sour-grapes attitude. So it is imperative to do away with the false imaginings of this "special being", namely, this unmanly or unwomanly self. That is sobering indeed, for then one will recognize that one is no different from *ordinary* men and women; the halo of superiority vanishes, and one understands that all this has boiled down to infantile inferiority complaints.

A man following this (self-)therapy will soon see through his role of not being manly. The role may express itself in small things, such as his conviction that he cannot stand alcohol. In reality, this is the unconscious role of the "tender boy" who is not up to such a tough habit. "Oh, but I really get sick after only one glass of whiskey!" is the likely reply. No, he makes himself believe that, and then, of course, he doesn't feel well, like a child who imagines he cannot stand some kinds of food but is not allergic at all. Shake off this role of sensitivity and try to enjoy a normal drink (only when you are so far along in growth that you might possibly consider abstinence, because only then will you be free to choose). "Alcoholic drinks are for *men*" is the false, near-hysterical view of many "child egos" in homosexual men. A "beautiful", "sweet", or narcissistic detail in one's dress, accentuating nonconformity with masculinity or "sensitivity", must be abolished in the same way. For men, effeminate shirts, showy rings or other ornaments, colognes, hairstyles, as well as one's way of speaking, the use of one's voice, gestures with fingers and hands, body movements, and gait must likewise be modified. It is instructive to listen to one's voice on a tape to discover unnatural, albeit unconscious, mannerisms that seem to proclaim: I am not manly (such as speaking slowly, with an affected, driveling, whining, or puling sound, which may irritate other people and which is so characteristic of certain homosexual men). After having studied your voice and perceived such particularities, try to speak quietly, but with a "sober", firm, and unaffected voice, and notice the difference (using a tape recorder). Also notice the resistance felt when doing this exercise.

Some lesbian women might do well to amend their stubborn aversion to wearing a nice gown or other typical women's dress. Use makeup, stop looking like a boy in his teens, and perhaps discover that then you will have to fight an emerging feeling of "being feminine is nothing for me". Try to mend a possibly ingrained playing of the role of the "hard fellow" with respect to your way of talking and intonation (listen to yourself on a tape), gesture and gait.

Little self-pampering habits must be changed, like that of the homosexual man who always brought his soft slippers when he went for a visit, because they "felt so comfortable to his feet" (a bit disrespectful to say, perhaps, but this is an example of being "old-womanish" or effeminate). Another man must stop excessively concentrating on his hobby of sewing, or arranging flowers, once he understands that he

enjoys such activities as a little child would, as a soft boy wallowing in his half-womanly "nature". Refraining from such
activities and hobbies once they have been detected as related
to the masculinity inferiority complex is frustrating. Com-
pare it, however, to the situation of the adolescent who understands that the time has come to go to bed without the
favorite teddy bear of childhood. Seek other activities and
amusement that lie more in the normal line and stir your
interest. The teddy bear example may perhaps make some
smile; all the same, many homosexuals inwardly do not want
to grow up; they cherish their childishness.

Once she discovers the connection to her "principled" rejection of "feminine" habits, a lesbian woman must break
through an aversion to cooking, for instance, or perhaps to
serving her guests, or, in another case, to devoting herself to
the so-called "unimportant" details of homemaking, to being
tender and *motherly* to small children, especially babies. (Contrary to what is often contended on the spurious basis of
pseudo-studies, some lesbian women are *inhibited* in their
motherly feelings and treat children as would adventurous
youth leaders rather than as mothers.) Abandoning themselves to the feminine "role" is a victory over their infantile
ego and at the same time an emotional revelation: a beginning of the experience of femininity.

Not infrequently, homosexual men must unlearn their
avoidance of getting their hands dirty doing manual work—
chopping wood, painting the house, using a shovel, a hammer. They must fight a resistance to physical effort. As to
sports, let the homosexual man, when the occasion offers itself, participate in a competitive game like soccer or baseball
and really try to do his best, even if he is anything but a star
on the field. And without self-pity; persevere and fight.
Some have afterward felt wonderful; a sportsmanlike fight—
meaning a victory over the "poor me" self—can make one

feel deeply that one is "a man". Normal gender-related activities are avoided, rejected, and fled from by the inner "child" in the homosexual; but my emphasis on the importance of taking on normal gender-linked "roles" is not the equivalent of "behavior therapy". For the important thing in making these changes is doing so with your *will*, in order to fight the inner resistance against these roles. Then it is not a question of training yourself as you would a monkey.

"Identifying" with one's manliness or womanliness by exercises in small everyday behaviors should not be exaggerated. Any attempt at showing off as "masculine", in hairstyles, mustaches, beards, showy "masculine" clothes, or the cultivation of muscles, is egocentric and childish and does nothing but feed the homosexual complex itself. Every affected person can list a number of behaviors and interests that for him must become points of attention.

Homosexual men often have a childish attitude toward physical pain, i.e., they "cannot stand" even relatively small physical hardships. Here we touch on the theme of *courage*, which is akin to *assertiveness*. The "inner child" is too fearful of both physical fighting and other forms of confrontation. His aggression therefore is often indirect, not open, and he may resort to intrigues and lying. To identify himself better with his masculinity, he must therefore fight his fear of confrontations, verbal and, if necessary, physical. He must speak his mind, honestly and frankly, defend himself if required by circumstances, and risk the aggression or ridicule of others. Further, he must exert authority if he is in the position of authority and not sidestep possible "attacks" of criticism by subordinates or colleagues. In trying to be normally assertive, he will come across his "poor me" child, and will have plenty of opportunity to hyperdramatize feelings of fear and of being a loser. Assertiveness is a good thing when our intelligence shows us that it is justified, even necessary, in certain situations. It can, however, be childish if its purpose is to demonstrate one's toughness and importance. Normal assertive behavior is quiet, rather than conspicuous, and effective.

Many lesbians, on the other hand, would greatly profit from small exercises in ordinary submissiveness, even—I hardly dare say the word!—in *obeying*; worse, in obeying the authority of *men*. Their preferred masculine role of dominance and independence must suffer some violence—exerted by themselves, by their own free will—if they are to *feel* what normal feminine "docility" and "softness" are. Generally a woman wants to live with the support of a man and to give herself to him, to care for him, and part of this is a longing to surrender to his masculinity. Below the spasmodic self-assertive behavior of the wounded "girl", this normal woman slumbers in every lesbian all the same.

One's body: the "unmanly boy" and "unfeminine girl" often have a rejective attitude, stemming from feelings of inferiority, toward the maleness or femaleness of their bodies. Try to accept fully and value positively your bodily maleness or femaleness. Look, for instance, at your naked self in the mirror and decide to be content with your manly or womanly body. Don't try compulsively to change some aspects of it by makeup or clothing, so that you no longer look the bodily type you are. If a woman has small breasts or is somewhat muscular, bony, and so forth, let her accept it, improve her appearance with reasonable limits, and, for the rest, stop complaining (this may be a repetitive exercise). The man should be glad and content with his physical type, with his penis, musculature, body hair, and so forth, and stop complaining about them or fantasizing about a different, so-called "ideal", physique. It is obvious that such dissatisfactions are infantile complaints!

10

RELATING TO OTHERS

Changing One's Views of and
Relationships with Others

The homosexual neurotic views others partly as a "child". To change homosexuality is hardly possible, if at all, without getting a more mature view of other people and a more adult way of relating to them.

Persons of the same sex

The homosexual must recognize the feelings of inferiority with respect to others of the same sex and of being ashamed among them, which are implicit in the idea of "not belonging". Combat such feeling by hyperdramatizing the poor inferior "child". It is advisable, furthermore, to take initiatives in making contacts rather than staying aloof or passive, to participate in conversations and activities, to invest energy in relating to others. These efforts will likely reveal a deeply ingrained habit of playing the role of the outsider, perhaps an aversion to adapt normally to others of the same sex, a negative view of others, a rejection of or indifference to them. The right motive for adapting better to others of the same sex is not, of course, the childish longing to be liked by them. In the first place, one must seek to *be* a good comrade oneself rather than to *have* one. That may mean a shift from a childish seeking for protection to taking responsibility for others.

From basic indifference toward another to trying to be interested in him. From infantile hostility, fear, and distrust to an attitude of sympathy and trust. From clinging and dependency to healthy inner independence. For homosexual men, this often means overcoming fears of confrontations, of criticism, and of aggression; and for lesbians, participating in womanly, perhaps motherly, interests and activities, as well as overcoming a certain contempt for them. Men often must lay aside their overcompliant, servile role, and women, their bossy, self-willed dominance.

A distinction must be made between individual and group contacts with same-sex contemporaries. Homosexually inclined persons often feel least at ease in same-sex groups of heterosexuals, especially when as children they had difficulties in adapting to same-sex groups, and in such situations experience feelings of inferiority. Here, especially, it will take courage to overcome group-avoidance behavior and comport oneself normally, naturally, without overcompensatory maneuvers, facing possible scorn or even ridicule, and yet behaving as simply one of the group.

Friendships

Normal friendships are a source of joy. In normal friendship, each person lives his life independently; there is neither the clinging dependence of the lonely "inner child" nor an ego-centered begging for attention. Building normal friendships, by "investing" interest in the other and not primarily in order to "get something in return", stimulates the process of emotional maturation. Besides, enjoyment of normal friendships with others of the same gender can stimulate the growth of gender identification; further, it counters loneliness complaints, which can so easily spur the self-comfort reactions of homosexual fantasy.

But then, a good, normal same-sex friendship may give

rise to an inner conflict. The homosexual may unwittingly slip into a childish idolization of his friend, and impulses of erotic yearning will present themselves. What is one to do in such a case? In general, it is better not to shun the friend. First, analyze the infantile element of your feelings and behavior with respect to him and counteract it by various methods, such as ceasing or changing certain behaviors—particularly, the habit of attracting his attention, protection, or care. Do not allow yourself any infantile enjoyment of his warmth for your poor person. Immediately put a stop to any fantasies in the erotic sphere (for instance, by hyper-dramatizing them). Take the firm resolution not to "betray" your friend by misusing him for childish lust, even if it be "only" in your imagination. Try to convert this strenuous situation into a challenge to grow up. See your friend's personality and physical appearance soberly, in real proportions: "He is not better than I am; both of us have positive as well as weak sides." Only if your infantile feelings for him threaten to overwhelm you, should you diminish the frequency of your contacts with him for a time. Without being scrupulous, avoid too great a physical intimacy, such as sleeping in one room. Most important: don't lean on his sympathy for you; fight off any impulse in that direction, for that would open the door to relapsing into your "child" personality.

One can systematically think over one's different relationships and make notes of specific interpersonal situations where infantile tendencies have to be combated and replaced by others more mature.

Older people

Homosexual men may look up to older men as if they were their fathers—fear their authority, be overly submissive to them, seek their protection, try to please them, or inwardly rebel against them. As always, first discover such attitudes in yourself and then try to replace them with new attitudes. Self-humor (e.g., hyperdramatizing your "little boy") and courage are beneficial here. Older women likewise may be viewed as a "mother" or an "aunt" to the homosexual man. His inner child may take on such roles as "the nice boy", "the servile boy", "the dependent, clinging boy", "the naughty boy" or "the enfant terrible" who perhaps does not openly go against his mother's wishes, yet constantly tries to revenge himself for her dominance over him in indirect ways, provoking her. "The pampered boy" childishly enjoys his mother's favoritism, protection, and indulgence. Such attitudes can be transferred to other women. Homosexual men who marry may transfer these attitudes to their wives and thus remain the "boy" who seeks pampering, protection, dominance, and support from a mother figure, and yet keep revenging themselves on her for her "dominance", real or spurious.

Homosexually inclined women may see (older) men as their fathers and transfer to them infantile aspects of the relationships with their own fathers. Men appear to them as disinterested, domineering, or far-away figures, or sometimes, depending on their situation in youth, as "buddies" "in the gang". Childhood reactions of rebellion, contempt, or special camaraderie are transferred from the father to other men. In some women, "masculine" self-affirming achievements are meant to satisfy their fathers' expectations. This can occur when a father unconsciously forced his daughter into the role of the "boy" achiever, esteeming her for that and not so much for her feminine qualities, or when, in the view of the adolescent girl, her father only esteemed the achievements of her brothers, so she started imitating the boy's role.

Parents

The "inner child" sticks to his infantile feelings, views, and behaviors, even if the parents are long dead. The homosexual man often remains fearful of, disinterested in, or rejective of his father, while at the same time seeking his approval. His attitude may be "I don't want to have anything to do with him" or "I don't take orders from him", if he views his father with contempt. He may remain his mother's "lovely boy", refusing to be grown-up in front of her as well as him. The path to take is twofold. First, accept your father as a father, and fight your aversion to him and your wish to take revenge on him. Instead, show him small signs of affection; begin to be interested in *his* life. Second, reject your mother's interference and/or her infantilizing you, firmly, but quietly; don't let yourself be "tyrannized" any more by her affections or anxious worries (if that is your case). Don't ask her advice too much or let her decide matters you should decide yourself. Your twofold aim is to untie a negative father-bonding as well as a "positive" mother-bonding. Become an independent, adult *son* to your parents, who treats them with special goodwill. Doing so will yield the reward of a more affectionate relationship with your father, with an increasing feeling of belonging to him, and possibly a somewhat more distant relationship with your mother, which will, however, be more authentic. Sometimes, a mother especially may object and try to restore the former infantile bonding, but in the end she usually will give in and the relationship will become less oppressive, more relaxed and normal. Don't be afraid of losing your mother or—in some cases—of some emotional blackmail on her part. You will have to "lead" your mother (but as a loving son) rather than the other way around.

Homosexually oriented women on their part often must fight their tendency to reject their mothers or at least toward a certain aversion or emotional resistance to her. Here too, it is a good method purposely to give her small tokens of affection, as a normally interested daughter would do. Above all, try to accept her, taking her difficult or unsympathetic traits for granted rather than reacting to them too dramatically. As is true for the male homosexual with regard to his father, try to *identify* with your mother's good qualities. The "inner child", in contradistinction, tends simply to reject everything coming from the parent whose affection it does not sufficiently experience. What in a parent cannot be objectively varnished over, one may distance oneself from, but that does not hinder a mature person from accepting and loving this same parent and accepting oneself as his or her child. After all, you are flesh of each one's flesh, you are of your parents' lineage. This sense of belonging to both of one's parents is a sign of emotional maturity.

Many lesbian women must liberate themselves from some imposed bonding with their fathers. Such a woman must learn not to give in to her father's wish to see and treat her as "male" company for himself or to achieve according to his expectations. She must shake off an imposed identification with him and instead have the attitude "I want to be the woman I really am, and as such be your *daughter*, not a kind of substitute son."

A "method" of great effectiveness in the struggle to make one's relations with one's parents more mature is to *forgive*. Often one cannot forgive at once. However, one can decide to forgive instantaneously in a concrete situation, for instance, at the moment one is thinking of certain behaviors and attitudes of one's parent(s). Forgiving is sometimes a struggle, but it normally gives relief and removes the blocks to normal and more loving feelings toward one's parents. In a way, it is synonymous with the attempt to stop inwardly complaining or pitying oneself about one's parent(s); but as forgiving also contains a moral dimension, its effect is likely to go deeper. But it does imply putting an end to one's self-pity. Forgiving is furthermore not a mere inner change of attitude. In order to be real, it must be materialized in gestures and small actions.

It is, however, not only a question of forgiving. If you see through your infantile attitudes toward your parents, you will see that you yourself, too, are responsible for some negative behaviors or for a lack of love for them. In changing your ways to them, sometimes by a clear "confession" or apology to them, you should also *ask* their *forgiveness* for yourself.

Changing Relations with the Opposite Sex; Marriage

The last step is the change from feeling and behaving like the "unmanly boy" or the "ungirlish girl" to feeling and behaving like a normal man or woman. The man must abolish his tendency to let himself be protected, pampered, or treated as a child by women (of his age) and/or his role of the "naïve brother among his sisters", of whom no manly dominance or manliness is required. Likewise, he must overcome his fear of women, the fear of the "pitiful child" who does not face up to the "man's role". Becoming a man means being able to take responsibility for and "lead" a woman. It means not letting oneself be dominated or led by a mother-woman, but, when appropriate, leading and making decisions for a woman himself. It is not exceptional that the initiative in the marriage of a homosexual man has come primarily from his wife, whereas the natural thing is for the man to win the woman. Normally, the woman wants to be won and desired by her beloved.

The woman with a homosexual complex has to fight her infantile resistance to surrender happily to her feminine role and to accept wholeheartedly the man's leading role. This is thought to be a sinful opinion by feminists, but, in fact, the ideology that obliterates sex roles is so unnatural that future generations will undoubtedly see it as a perversion of a decadent culture. Male-female role differences are inborn, and persons who fight their homosexual tendencies have to return to them.

Heterosexual feelings come only in the wake of restored feelings of manliness or womanliness. There should be no "training" in heterosexuality, however, for that would feed the inferior self-image: "I have to *prove* my manliness (or womanliness)." So, before entering into a more intimate relationship with a person of the opposite sex, one should have fallen in love, including having an erotic attraction. For a recovering homosexual, sometimes—not as a rule, however—several years may pass by before he reaches this point. Yet in general it is better to wait than to commence prematurely a marriage relationship. Marriage is not the direct goal of the battle for sexual normality; it should not be artificially or spasmodically set as a target.

Not a few committed homosexuals enviously hate marriage and become furious when one of their heterosexual friends becomes engaged to marry. They actually feel excluded and inferior, and insofar as they are "children" or "teenagers", they do not understand much of the male-female relationship. Progressing out of their neurosis, however, homosexually inclined people gradually, or by fits and starts, become aware of the male-female dynamic and do away with their resistance to the idea that this male-female world of the "adults" could also be something "*for me*".

In conclusion: never abuse another to affirm your already growing heterosexual orientation. If a romantic affair is sought merely to prove one's (developing) heterosexuality, there is a real risk of being thrown back into one's former infantilisms. Do not start an intimate relationship until it has become clear that there is real mutual love, including but beyond erotic attraction, and to such a degree that both have decided to be faithful. That is, you then choose the other person for his *own* sake.

BIBLIOGRAPHY

Adler, A. 1930. Das Problem der Homosexualität (The problem of homosexuality). *Zeitschrift der Individualpsychologie*. Beiheft 1.

Alan Guttmacher Institute. 1993. The sexual behavior of men in the U.S. *Family Planning Perspectives* 25:52–62.

Arndt, J. L. 1961. Ein bijdrage tot het inzicht in de homoseksualiteit (A contribution to the understanding of homosexuality). *Geneeskundige Bladen* 3:65–105.

Bailey, J. M., and R. C. Pillard. 1991. A genetic study of male sexual orientation. *Archives of General Psychiatry* 48:1089–96.

Baldwin, J. 1985. *The price of the ticket*. London: Joseph Michael.

Baruk, H. 1979. *Menschen wie Wir* (*Men like we are*). Düsseldorf/Vienna: Econ Verlag.

Bell, A. P., and M. S. Weinberg. 1978. *Homosexualities: a study of diversity among men and women*. New York: Simon & Schuster.

Bergler, E. 1957. *Homosexuality: Disease or way of life?* New York: Hill & Wang.

Byne, W. 1994. The biological evidence challenged. *Scientific American* 270:26–31.

Byne, W., and B. Parsons. 1993. Human sexual orientation. *Archives of General Psychiatry* 50:228–39.

Cameron, P., et al. 1991. *The life span of homosexuals*. Washington: Family Research Institute.

Cameron, P. 1992. *Medical consequences of what homosexuals do*. Washington: Family Research Institute.

———. 1993. *The gay nineties*. Franklin, Tenn.: Adroit Press.

————. 1994. *The truth about "gay parents"*. Washington: Family Research Institute.

Dannecker, M. 1978. *Der Homosexuelle und die Homosexualität (The homosexual and homosexuality)*. Frankfurt: Syndikat.

Escrivá de Balaguer, J. 1988. *The forge*. New Rochelle, N.Y.: Scepter Press.

Fenichel, O. 1945. *The psychoanalytic theory of neurosis*. New York: Norton.

Ferenczi, S. 1950. The nosology of male homosexuality—Homoeroticism. In: *Contributions to Psychoanalysis*. New York: Brunner-Mazel (original article 1914).

Frankl, V. 1975. Paradoxical intention and dereflection. *Psychotherapy: Theory, Research and Practice* 12:226–37.

Green, R. 1985. Gender identity in childhood and later sexual orientation: Follow-up of 75 males. *American Journal of Psychiatry* 142:339–41.

————. 1987. *The "sissy boy syndrome" and the development of homosexuality*. New Haven/London: Yale University Press.

Gundlach, R. H., and B. F. Riess. 1967. Birth order and sex of siblings in a sample of lesbians and nonlesbians. *Psychological Reports* 20:61–62.

Hamer, D. H., S. Hu, V. L. Magnuson, N. Hu, and A. M. L. Pattatucci. 1993. A linkage between DNA markers on the X chromosome and male sexual orientation. *Science* 261:321–27.

Hanson, D. 1965. *Homosexuality: The international disease*. New York: L. S. Publications.

Harris, T. A. 1973. *I'm OK, you're OK*. London: Pan Books.

Harvey, J. F. 1987. *The homosexual person*. San Francisco: Ignatius Press.

————. 1996. *The truth about homosexuality: The cry of the faithful*. San Francisco: Ignatius Press.

Hatterer, L. J. 1980. *The pleasure addicts*. South Brunswick/ New York: Barnes & Yoseloff.

Herink, R., ed. 1980. *The psychotherapy handbook*. New York: The New American Library.

Hockenberry, S. L., and R. E. Billingham. 1987. Sexual orientation and boyhood gender conformity: Development of the boyhood gender conformity scale. *Archives of Sexual Behavior* 16:475–87.

Horney, K. 1950. *Neurosis and inner growth*. New York: Norton.

Howard, J. 1991. *Out of Egypt*. Speldhurst, Kent: Monarch Publications.

Isay, R. A. 1989. *Being homosexual: Gay men and their development*. Harmondsworth: Penguin.

Janssens, G. J. B. A. 1939. Medisch-psychiatrische beschouwingen en therapie der homosexualiteit (Medical-psychiatric observations and therapy of homosexuality) in *Het vraagstuk der homosexualiteit* (*The problem of homosexuality*). Roermond: Romen.

Kallmann, F. J. 1952. Comparative twin studies on the genetic aspects of male homosexuality. *Journal of Nervous and Mental Disease* 115:283–89.

Korver, H., and R. Govaars. 1988. Laatste biecht van ein drugsplayboy (Last confession of a drugs playboy). *De Telegraaf* (July 23).

Lejeune, J. 1993. Letter to the author (November 27).

LeVay, S. 1991. A difference in hypothalamic structure between heterosexual and homosexual men. *Science* 253:1034–37.

McWhirter, D. P., and A. M. Mattison. 1984. *The male couple: How relationships develop*. Englewood Cliffs, N.J.: Prentice-Hall.

Missildine, W. H. 1963. *Your inner child of the past*. New York: Simon & Schuster.

Mohr, J. W., R. E. Turner, and M. B. Jerry. 1964. *Pedophilia and exhibitionism: A handbook*. Toronto: University of Toronto Press.

Murray, H. A. 1953. *Explorations in personality*. New York: Oxford University Press.

Nicolosi, J. 1991. *Reparative therapy of male homosexuality*. Northvale, N.J./London: Jason Aronson.

Risch, N., E. Squires-Wheeler, and B. J. B. Keats. 1993. Male sexual orientation and genetic evidence. *Science* 262:2063–64.

Rogers, C. R. 1951. *Client-centered therapy*. Boston: Houghton.

Schnabel, P. 1993. De ontwikkeling van de mannelijke homoseksualiteit volgens psychoanalyticus Richard A. Isay (The development of male homosexuality according to Richard A. Isay). *Nieuwe Rotterdamsche Courant* (July 24).

Schofield, M. 1965. *The sexual behaviour of young people*. London: Little, Brown & Company.

Siering, U. 1988. *Männliche Identität und Initiation im erzählerischen Werk von James Baldwin* (*Male identity and initiation in the stories of James Baldwin*). Thesis. Kassel.

Stampfl, T. G., and D. J. Levis. 1967. Essentials of implosive therapy. *Journal of Abnormal Psychology* 72:496–503.

Stekel, W. 1922. *Psychosexueller Infantilismus* (Psychosexual infantilism). Vienna: Urban & Schwarzenberg.

Stern, K. 1951. *The pillar of fire*. New York: Harcourt, Brace & Company.

Stoller, R. J., and G. H. Herdt. 1985. Theories of origins of male homosexuality. *Archives of General Psychiatry* 42:399–404.

van den Aardweg, G. J. M. 1965. De neurose van Couperus (The neurosis of Couperus). *Nederlands Tijdschrift voor de Psychologie* 20:293–307.

———. 1984. Parents of homosexuals: Not guilty? *American Journal of Psychotherapy* 38:180–89.

————. 1985. *Homosexuality and hope.* Ann Arbor, Mich.: Servant Publications.

————. 1986. *On the origins and treatment of homosexuality: A psychoanalytic reinterpretation.* New York: Praeger.

Van Lennep, D. J., A. C. Rümke, and R. H. Houwink. 1954. *Report on a study of a number of overt homosexual male and female subjects.* Utrecht: Rijks Universiteit, Institute of Clinical Psychology.

Wellings, K., et al. 1994. *Sexual behaviour in Britain.* Harmondsworth: Penguin.

Wilson, J. Q. 1993. *The moral sense.* New York: The Free Press.

INDEX